Falls Assessment and Prevention

HOME, HOSPICE, AND EXTENDED CARE

Falls Assessment and Prevention

HOME, HOSPICE, AND EXTENDED CARE

Lynn S. Alvord, Ph.D.

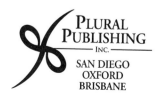

PLURAL
PUBLISHING
INC.
SAN DIEGO
OXFORD
BRISBANE

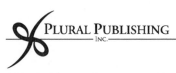

PLURAL PUBLISHING
INC.

5521 Ruffin Road
San Diego, CA 92123
e-mail: info@pluralpublishing.com
Web site: http://www.pluralpublishing.com

49 Bath Street
Abingdon, Oxfordshire OX14 1EA
United Kingdom

Typeset in 11/13 Garamond by Flanagan's Publishing Services, Inc.
Printed in the United States of America by McNaughton and Gunn

Library of Congress Cataloging-in-Publication Data:

Alvord, Lynn Stephen, 1949-
  Falls assessment and prevention : home, hospital, and extended care /
Lynn S. Alvord.
      p. ; cm.
  Includes bibliographical references.
  ISBN-13: 978-1-59756-120-4 (alk. paper)
  ISBN-10: 1-59756-120-7 (alk. paper)
  1. Falls (Accidents) in old age. I. Title.
  [DNLM: 1. Accidental Falls—prevention & control. 2. Aged. WA 288
A476f 2007]
  RD93.5.A35A48 2007
  613.6'9—dc22
                                                                2007050051

Contents

Preface

This book is intended as a resource and text for those of varied professions as well as the public who are involved in the prevention of falls. The overriding goal of the book is to present not only current information, but to introduce original ideas in the area of falls prevention. For example, a new falls screening tool based upon a medical model for falls assessment is presented. Whereas previous measures select a limited set of risk factors to assess, the new tool presented draws from outcome studies of our medically based Falls Prevention Clinic, a multi-specialty outpatient clinic at Henry Ford Hosptal in Detroit, Michigan. At the time of this writing, the outcome data on the effectiveness of this multi-specialty clinic are being presented in an upcoming article in the journal, Ear, Nose and Throat, demonstrating a high rate of success of the clinic for reducing falls. Also presented in the book is a new behavior based walking method, called "SafeWalk," aimed at teaching the falling patient new safe habits for walking and turning. These content features of the book reflect our philosophy, that falling is as much a "behavioral" issue as it is a medical one. The book is also intended to develop the topic into a true "science" by analyzing the theoretical aspects of falling and its prevention. Also included are chapters on the science of balance and mobility, specific coverage of setting up a "falls prevention clinic, a theory of falling, prevention measures, risk factors, and case studies to illustrate the concepts covered. The core conviction of the author is that most falls can be prevented if correct principles are coupled with adequate personal motivation. Considering ie dire consequences of the falling and its impact on individuals 'quering this problem is well worth the ongoing efforts of al' se who are involved in falls prevention.

Introduction

The Secret Fallers

Zelma, my 92-year-old mother, lives with us in our home. She is in relatively good health, but is frail and has osteoporosis. Zelma is pleasant, does some of her own cooking and cleaning, and dresses herself every day, complete with the small heeled dress shoes she has worn all her life. Although she broke a hip 4 years ago due to a fall, luckily her recovery was rapid and complete. One night not too long ago my wife and I were sitting in the basement watching television. We suddenly heard a thud above us that sounded like someone had thrown a sack of potatoes on the floor. After exchanging a brief look of dread with my wife, I ran up the stairs to find Zelma in her bedroom just getting up from a fall. With a sheepish smile on her face, she said, "I wasn't going to tell you that I fell." This made me wonder how many previous falls she had had while living alone.

In our clinic, the prevalence of older fallers who are keeping their falls a secret is high. Perhaps out of fear of losing their independence, having to go to the doctor, or being required to use a cane or walker, such frequent fallers often are not seen by a doctor until a major injury has occurred. These "secret fallers" will often finally come in with bruises, scrapes or worse, or will attend our clinic because they have been caught falling by a relative who has noticed several falls or near misses recently. Alone with the patient in the exam room, people will often confide in us about their falls once trust has been established. We never ask the simple question "*have* you fallen?" Rather, we always phrase the question this way, "In the past six months, *how many times* have you fallen?" The answers are sobering as these patients reply with answers such as, "six," "ten," or even "thirty times." Weekly or even daily falls are frequently reported. Obviously, there is an element of denial during the first period of falling in which the person is not yet willing to admit a problem or is not yet certain that there is a problem. After admitting their falls in our clinic, patients will sometimes ask that we not tell their relative in the waiting room about the falls. In addition to falling, patients will also sometimes admit other dangerous or sad behaviors such as climbing the stairs on hands and knees, rushing to the bathroom several times per night, or not bathing frequently for fear of falling in the tub or shower. Such revelations dispel the myth of the "one big fall" in which the aging person breaks a hip. Because most persons we evaluate have had several falls but with only minor injuries, we believe that it is typical for several falls to occur before the fall causing a major injury. With the high incidence of falls in older adults over the age of 80, it is probably safe to just assume that falls are occurring more and more frequently in a given aging individual. The principles in this book could therefore be applied almost universally to those of advancing age.

This book has one major premise, which is that through a combination of medical assessment, education, and prevention measures, **most falls can be prevented**. Studies show that falls can be successfully reduced using interventions such as adding home safety features, providing education, medical intervention, exercise or assistive walking equipment. A variety of falls prevention clinics, outreach programs, and medical interventions also have been shown to be effective. The jury is still out as to the optimum method for the majority of people; in fact, there is recognition that customizing falls prevention measures for a specific individual is usually necessary. One thing is clear from the research, falls can be prevented in many individuals. Safety from falls provides a much needed element of safety, freedom, and independence to the lives of aging individuals as well as other fallers. For falls prevention to be effective, **three building blocks of falls prevention are needed: medical assessment, behavioral change**, and **falls education**. Each of these elements will be discussed in the first chapter and elsewhere in the book. The book emphasizes the practical techniques needed to reduce the risk of falls and their injuries. Many of the ideas and techniques outlined in this book have been developed through working with hundreds of fall-prone individuals attending the balance laboratory and Falls Prevention Clinic at Henry Ford Hospital.

Organization of the Book

In order that this book may be a useful resource for the expert as well as the general public, the material within chapters is organized so that the more general information having common interest is presented first, with the more specific and technical information found toward the end of each chapter.

Summary

In summary, although falls are becoming more prevalent in our aging society, there is hope for significant improvement in falls prevention through proper medical assessment, establishing appropriate behavioral changes, and providing education for care providers as well as potential fallers.

CHAPTER 1

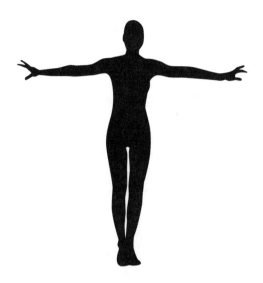

Scope of the Problem—
Hope for Solutions

The premise of this book is that most falls can be prevented through appropriate medical intervention, behavioral changes, and education. This chapter outlines the "falls problem" in terms of various "**costs**" to the individual and society, provides **information about current efforts** directed toward solving the problem, and describes **a basic philosophy** for falls prevention.

"Costs" to the Individual

Although falls can cause injury at any age, they are most dangerous among the aging population. Sadly for the older adult, falls begin to happen just when the aging person is more susceptible to injury. In babies and toddlers, bones are not yet fully ossified or brittle; therefore, falls, which are a rather common occurrence, rarely cause injury. In the older adult, just the opposite is the case. In the aging adult, who may have osteoporosis, lack of strength sufficient to cushion a fall, or slowed reaction times, the effects of a fall are often devastating.

The following statistics emphasize the scope of the problem. Falls play a major role in mortality, morbidity, and hospitalization in older individuals (Mayo, Vlahov, Myers, & Al-Ibrahim, 1990; Korner-Bitensky et al., 1989; Nyberg & Gustafson, 1995). Approximately 30% of community dwelling older individuals (over age 65) fall every year (Gillespie, Gillespie et al., 2001). In a study by Josephson, Fabacher, and Rubenstein (1991), falls injuries were found to be the fifth leading cause of death in the elderly; however, in another study, falls and "other significant adverse events" were listed as the seventh leading cause of death among the elderly (Desai & Zhang, 1999). Among the older population, falling has also been cited as the most common cause of nonfatal injuries and hospitalizations for trauma (Alexander, Rivara, & Wolf, 1992), with nearly 8% of persons age 70 or over visiting emergency rooms every year for an injury incurred by a fall (Sattin et al., 1990). Of these, approximately one-third are admitted to the hospital (Grisso et al., 1992; Sattin, 1992).

These and similar statistics emphasize the impact of falls on older individuals. However, falls not only affect the aging population but can also pose significant health risks at any age especially for those with neuromuscular or other chronic disorders affecting balance or mobility. For example, falls are a leading cause of traumatic brain injury among those admitted to emergency rooms (Jager, Weiss, Coben, & Pepe, 2000).

Death and Injury

There is disagreement as to what percentage of falls causes injury. It has long been the perception that "grandma will fall, and when she does, she will break her hip." In a recent survey among our patients at the Henry Ford Hospital Falls Prevention Clinic, we found that approximately one-third had fallen three or more times in the previous six months, most without serious injury. Another study in 2001 by Gillespie, Gillespie, et al. showed that fewer than 1 in 10 falls resulted in fracture, although approximately 20% of all falls required medical attention (Gillespie, Gillespie, et al., 2001). According to a study by Nevitt, Cummings, and Hudes (1991), most falls resulted in minor soft tissue injuries (bruises and scrapes), with 10 to 15% of falls resulting in fractures.

Death rates resulting from falls have also been studied. In a large epidemiologic study, Sattin, Huber, DeVito, et al. (1990) reported a death rate of 2.2% among elderly patients seeking emergency care after an injurious fall. Although this number seems low, **eventual complications can also lead to death**. Deaths from falls complications are a leading cause of death from injury in those above age 65 and the greater the age, the higher the death rate attributable to falls. The highest death rate is in white men over the age of 85, with 180 deaths per 100,000 (Sattin, 1992). As stated above, in the previously mentioned study by Josephson, Fabacher, and Rubenstein (1991), falls injuries were found to be the fifth leading cause of death in the elderly. Only strokes, cancers, and lung and heart disorders were higher (Josephson et al., 1991).

Psychological Costs

One underrated consequence of falls is the possible adverse psychological effect on the individual. Although injury from falls such as a broken hip is no longer a death sentence, mainly due to improved surgical and rehabilitative methods, many older individuals consider such an event as "the beginning of the end." Much educational effort is needed to apprise the public of the fact that falling or even breaking a hip is no longer a "death sentence." Still, the psychological impact of falls is very detrimental to a significant number of individuals. **Fear of falling** is one such psychological result of a fall that has negative consequences. Those who fall are more likely to become fearful of future falls (Tinetti, Mendes de Leon, Doucette, & Baker, 1994). The so-called "**post-fall anxiety syndrome**" is a well-recognized problem often resulting in a loss of confidence to walk safely. Such fears may result in self-imposed functional limitations. Even more striking was a study showing that

80% of elderly women reported preferring death over a "bad" hip fracture that may cause them to have to enter a nursing home (Salkeld, Cameron, Cumming, et al., 2000). This seems to show that the perception of injury is sometimes a significant problem in itself.

Nursing Home Placement After Falls

Falls are associated with an increased likelihood of being placed in a nursing home (Donald & Bulpitt, 1999; Grisso, Schwarz, & Wolfson, et al., 1992). Tinnetti and Williams (1997) studied a group of 133 fallers, some of whom had experienced injuries. Twelve percent of the group was admitted to a long-term nursing home stay. When adjusted for other risk factors, fallers having at least one injurious fall had a relative risk of 10.2 of being admitted compared to those having no falls (were ten times more likely to be admitted than nonfallers). Another study found that falls were a major reason for 40% of nursing home admissions (Bezon, Echevarria, & Smith, 1999). Once in a nursing home, however, falls often do not cease. It has been estimated that approximately half of those in long-term care settings will eventually fall.

Other Declines After Falls

Declines in various other abilities or functions are also seen more often after falls. (Kiel, O'Sullivan, Teno, & Mor, 1991; Tinetti, Mendes de Leon, Doucette, & Baker, 1994; Tinetti & Williams, 1998). Those unable to get up after a fall by themselves also often suffer other lasting declines (Tinetti, Liu, & Claus, 1993). Increased use of medical services, decrease in basic activities of daily living, and decline in social and physical activity are all consequences seen more frequently after falls. In their study, Tinetti, Liu, and Claus (1993) reported, in the *Journal of the American Medical Association*, that many older individuals who fall are unable to help themselves up (about half), resulting in the "**long lie**," that is, lying on the floor for hours before being discovered.

Falls generally recur. Nearly 60% of those who have already fallen will fall again (Nevitt, Cummings, & Hudes, 1991).

Unaware of Risks

There is evidence from past studies that many elderly individuals who fall are unaware of the risks of falling and often do not recognize nor report risk factors to physicians (Cumming, Kelsey, & Nevitt, 1990; Cummings, Nevitt, & Kidd, 1988; Jarrett, Rockwood, Carver, et al., 1995). It is also likely that many older individuals do not recall and report with accuracy the details of their falls.

"Costs" to Society

Financial costs to society from falls are tremendous. In addition to the costs of research and falls prevention programs, the medical costs to the health care system are substantial. Hip fractures alone are very costly, contributing the single largest expense of the approximate $20 billion in direct medical costs attributed to all fall-related injuries in 2000 (U.S. Department of Health and Human Services, 2003). In the state of Washington alone, in 1989, of the nearly one billion dollars in total hospital charges, approximately 5% ($53,346,191) were attributable to charges for fall-related trauma (Alexander, Rivara, & Wolf, 1992).

Current Efforts

Many government and health care agencies are recognizing the magnitude of the falls problem as outlined in the previous section and are promoting research studies, falls prevention programs, and educational materials in a widespread effort to arrive at solutions. Many of the references in this book come from these governmental efforts. One example of a successful government sponsored effort is "Falls Free." In 2005, the National Council on Aging, the Archstone Foundation, and the Home Safety Council collaborated in the initiative, "Falls Free: Promoting a National Falls Prevention Action Plan" (National Council on Aging Web Site, 2007). The goal of the initiative was to provide information that would aid the public, those working in health care services, and those working in home construction to become more knowledgeable and aware of falls problems so that solutions could be found. The National Council on Aging provides an excellent Web site where current research findings and additional information can be found (see Falls Free at National Council on Aging's Web site, http://www.ncoa.org/con tent.cfm?sectionID=105&detail=902).

Working Toward a Solution

Falls prevention requires effort in the following three areas: *Medical assessment* in order to understand and treat underlying causes of falls and reverse those causes if possible; *Behavioral changes* that will result in safer habits and practices; and *education* of both fall-prone individuals and their families and caretakers. These three areas are each addressed in later sections of the book, but are briefly discussed here (Figure 1-1).

Medical Assessment

Although falling is often primarily a behavioral problem, or at least can be controlled behaviorally (see below), in our experience, one or more medical abnormalities are present in those who fall frequently. The causes of falls are so varied that **individual assessment** and recommendations are necessary to effectively prevent falls. The medical problem may be a major disorder such as a seizure or cardiovascular abnormality, or may be quite minor such as pain in the feet. In reality, many older individuals have more than one medical problem contributing to falls (multifactorial). Also, it is often a combination of a medical and a behavioral factor that leads

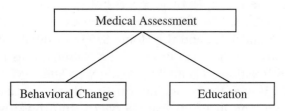

Figure 1-1. The three key elements of falls prevention.

to falls. For example, if a person has a relatively minor medical problem that could lead to falls, such as borderline visual acuity, and then combines that disorder with the tendency to rush, there is a much higher likelihood of falling.

In short, the need for medical assessment is critical to the prevention of falls in fall-prone individuals. Often, such medical evaluations uncover two or more minor problems that, when combined, cause falls, such as poor vision and muscle weakness. On the other hand, it is possible for a single serious medical condition to cause falls, even in a younger patient. Because of the combination of causal factors, various multidisciplinary efforts have been initiated, based either on a medical or community health service model. There is evidence that multidisciplinary programs can be effective (Chang et al., 2004; Close et al., 1999). In our opinion, the most effective medically based "falls assessment clinic" is one that considers all body systems capable of causing falls, uses a team approach, and provides appropriate intervention such as physical or occupational therapy, as well as outreach exercise programs. We describe our Falls Prevention Clinic, at Henry Ford Hospital, later in the book.

Behavioral Changes

With adequate behavioral changes alone, most falls can be prevented despite the medical factors leading to falls. This is a bold statement; however, as we work with fall-prone individuals, it becomes apparent that falling is usually a combination of behavioral and medical problems. Very often, falls occur when "at risk" persons push their limits doing something a little out of the ordinary such as carrying something while using the stairs, hurrying to a phone that has been misplaced, using a step stool, or rushing to the bathroom. Although many dizzy persons instinctively make their home less dangerous by placing objects such as furniture in the middle of rooms that can serve as walking aids, certain personality types will not sacrifice appearance for safety. For that matter, many people find it difficult to change very much about themselves or their environment for the sake of safety, such as slowing their rapid walking style or storing things at a lower level. Other dangerous actions leading to falls may be performed in ignorance or simply out of habit. The good news is that even someone who is knowingly participating in a dangerous activity may not necessarily shun a useful newer safe technique when one is presented. Most fallers are unaware of the newer techniques such as those presented in this book (see Chapter 6). We are all creatures of habit and many fallers are individuals who have built habits both good and bad over many years. Still, many studies have shown that falls can be prevented, which emphasizes the need for behavioral modification as well as medical intervention in falls prevention. Our philosophy is that as good habits and techniques are learned, these can more easily replace the old habits. We address the subject of introducing new, safer habits of ambulation in a later chapter.

Education

Knowledge is extremely valuable to the potential faller. For example, I often receive surprised looks from patients when I inform them that, based on testing, they are apt to have a much harder time keeping their balance in the dark due to an inner ear balance disorder. Knowing their individual strengths and weaknesses gives patients more freedom because they can do simple things to improve their balance such as use more lighting, perform simple exercises, or change their footwear.

The fear of falling is itself one of the most significant falls risk factors. Education can often help the patient overcome unwarranted fears. Such fear may prevent a person from exercising, which leads to decreased muscle strength and increased falls risk. Educating the potential faller about his or her strengths promotes confidence, which, in turn, leads to increased levels of activity and reduced falls risk.

Because many fall-prone individuals are aging, the question is: "Can older individuals really develop new habits of increased activity and safety that can lead to reduced falls?" The answer is "yes," but the learning process takes time. A person at age 70 requires more time to learn new skills and habits than a person in their twenties. Many aging individuals have a surprising capacity to adapt to new skills and mental demands but adjusting to new ideas usually takes longer than it once did. In dealing with older individuals, often into their nineties, we should not expect changes in behaviors to come too quickly, let alone within a single lecture or counseling session. Habits developed over a lifetime are very hard to break. For example, we cannot expect to teach a person in their nineties in 2 weeks to stop using the step stool that has been used for decades. On the other hand, older individuals often demonstrate an amazing capacity for learning new things. A woman in her late seventies known to the author joined a gym and learned to swim, a skill she had always wanted to obtain. But the same older woman found it hard to break certain old habits. Therefore, it is easier to learn new techniques such as safer ways of walking than to try to break old habits. More about behavior modification is presented later in the book.

Education is vital not only to the potential faller, but to the family, caretaker, and health care professional. This book emphasizes the information necessary to empower both the potential faller as well as those professionals who hope to prevent falls. This information includes not only techniques for safer mobility, but also a look at available equipment designed to help those having mobility problems.

Summary

In summary, the costs of falls and their associated injuries are extremely high, both for society as well as individual patients. Efforts in falls prevention should focus on **medical assessment**, **behavioral modification**, and **education**. This book examines each of these areas in detail with the conviction that most falls can be prevented if these elements are accompanied by adequate patient motivation.

References

Alexander, B. H., Rivara, F. P., & Wolf, M. E. (1992). The cost and frequency of hospitalization for fall-related injuries in older adults. *American Journal of Public Health, 82*(7), 1020–1023.

Bezon, J., Echevarria, K. H., & Smith, G. B. (1999). Nursing outcome indicator: Preventing falls for elderly people. *Outcomes Management for Nursing Practice, 9*(3), 112–116.

Chang, J. T., Morton, S. C., Rubenstein, L. Z., Mojica, W. A., Maglione, M., Suttorp, M., et al. (2004). Interventions for the prevention of falls in older adults: Systematic review and meta-analysis of randomized clinical trials. *British Medical Journal, 328*(7441), 680–683.

Close, J., Ellis, M., Hooper, R., Glucksman, E., Jackson, S., & Swift, C. (1999). Prevention of falls in the elderly trial (PROFET): A randomized controlled trial. *Lancet, 353*(7441), 93–97.

Cumming, R. G., Kelsey, J. L., & Nevitt, M. C. (1990). Methodologic issues in the study of frequent and recurrent health problems. Falls in the elderly. *Annals of Epidemiology, 1*, 49–56.

Cummings, S. R., Nevitt, M. C., & Kidd, S. (1988). Forgetting falls: The limited accuracy of recall of falls in the elderly. *Journal of the American Geriatric Society, 36*, 613–616.

Desai, M. M, Zhang, P., & Hennessy, C. H. (1999). Surveillance for morbidity and mortality among older adults—United States, 1995–1996. *Mortality Morbidity Weekly Report, 48*(8), 7–25.

Donald, I. P., & Bulpitt, C. J. (1999). The prognosis of falls in elderly people living at home. *Age and Ageing, 28*, 121–125.

Gillespie, L. D., Gillespie, W. J., et al. (2001). Interventions for preventing falls in elderly people. *Cochrane Review.* (Cochrane Database Syst Rev 3: CD000340.)

Grisso, J. A., Schwarz, D. F., Wolfson, V., Polansky, M., LaPann K., et al. (1992). The impact of falls in an inner-city African-American population. *Journal of the American Geriatric Society, 40*, 673–678.

Jager, T. E., Weiss, H. B., Coben, J. H., & Pepe, P. E. (2000). Traumatic brain injuries evaluated in U.S. emergency departments, 1992–1994. *Academic Emergency Medicine, 7*(2), 134–140.

Jarrett, P.G., Rockwood, K., Carver, D., Stolee, P, & Cosway, S. (1995). Illness presentation in elderly patients. *Archives of Internal Medicine, 155*, 1060–1064.

Josephson, K. R., Fabacher, D. A., & Rubenstein, L. Z. (1991). Home safety and fall prevention. *Clinical Geriatric Medicine, 7*, 707–731.

Kiel, D. P., O'Sullivan, P., Teno, J. M., & Mor, V. (1991). Health care utilization and functional status in the aged following a fall. *Medical Care, 29*(3), 221–228.

Mayo, N. E., Korner-Bitensky, N., Becker, R., & Georges P. (1989). Predicting falls among patients in a rehabilitation hospital. *American Journal of Physical Medicine and Rehabilitation, 68*, 139–146.

National Council on Aging. (2007). Falls free: Promoting a national falls prevention plan. Web site: http://www.ncoa.org/content.cfm?sectionID=10 5&detail=902

Nevitt, M. C., Cummings, S. R., & Hudes, E. S. (1991). Risk factors for injurious falls: A prospective study. *Journal of Gerontology, 46*(5), M164–M170.

Nyberg, L., & Gustafson, Y. (1995). Patient falls in stroke rehabilitation. A challenge to rehabilitation strategies. *Stroke, 26,* 838-842.

Salkeld, G., Cameron, I. D., Cumming, R. G., Easter, S., Seymour, J., Kurrle, S. E., & Ouine, S. (2000). Quality of life related to fear of falling and hip fracture in older women: A time trade off study. *British Medical Journal, 320*(7231), 341-346.

Sattin, R. W. (1992). Falls among older persons: A public health perspective. *Annual Revue of Public Health, 13,* 489-508.

Sattin, R. W., Lambert Huber, D. A., DeVito, C. A., Rodriguez, J. G., Ros, A., Bacchelli, S., et al. (1990). The incidence of fall injury events among the elderly in a defined population. *American Journal of Epidemiology, 131*(6), 1028-1037.

Tinetti, M. E., Liu, W. L., & Claus, E. B. (1993). Predictors and prognosis of inability to get up after falls among elderly persons. *Journal of the American Medical Association, 269*(1), 65-70.

Tinetti, M. E., Mendes de Leon, C. F., Doucette, J. T., & Baker, D. I. (1994). Fear of falling and fall-related efficacy in relationship to functioning among community-living elders. *Journal of Gerontology, 49*(3), M140-M147.

Tinetti, M. E., & Williams, C. S. (1997). Falls, injuries due to falls, and the risk of admission to a nursing home. *New England Journal of Medicine, 337*(18), 1279-1284.

Tinetti, M. E., & Williams, C. S. (1998). The effect of falls and fall injuries on functioning in community-dwelling older persons. *Journals of Gerontology Series A: Biological Sciences and Medical Sciences, 53*(2), M112-M119.

U.S. Department of Health and Human Services. (2003). *Falls prevention interventions in the Medicare population. Evidence report and evidence-based recommendations.* Prepared by the RAND Corporation, Santa Monica, California.

Vlahov, D., Myers, A. H., & Al-Ibrahim, M. S. (1990). Epidemiology of falls among patients in a rehabilitation hospital. *Archives of Physical and Medical Rehabilitation, 71,* 8-12.

CHAPTER 2

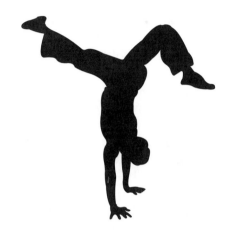

Balance and Mobility

We need both **balance** and **mobility** in order to stand and walk safely without falling. This chapter deals with the physiologic components of balance, gait, and mobility including common abnormalities affecting these functions.

The Balance System

There are three basic "balance systems": **vestibular, somatosensory**, and **visual**. Because these interact and are coordinated in the brainstem it may be argued that these three are really components of one single "balance system." The vestibular system, often too simply referred to as the "inner ear or labrynthine balance system," actually consists of systems outside the ear including several subsystems interconnecting to the neck (cervicovestibular), cerebellum, and arms and legs (vestibulospinal tract). The somatosensory system refers to sensors in the muscles and joints of the lower extremities allowing for determination of the position of the limbs. Pressure receptors or "proprioceptors" are found primarily in the joints and muscles. The visual balance system refers not only to vision, but also to the eye's ability to move smoothly and accurately (oculomotor function). As to which of these three balance systems is the most important, the argument continues because each has its own special function and strengths. However, if we ask, "which of these can we 'not do without,'" the answer would need to be the "somatosensory" system. Evidence for this is that those who have lost both their vision and their inner ear balance function can still usually keep their balance to a degree having only their somatosensory system intact.

Loss of function in any one of these three systems (Table 2–1), vestibular, somatosensory, or visual, can result in imbalance or falls. For example, one of the most common types of falls occurs when we simply do not sense that we are tipping until it is too late. This can occur with even minor impairments of the balance system. When tipping off balance, a leg needs to move quickly to catch the body before falling. Unfortunately, many older persons have minor deficits not only in their balance sense, but also in their ability to quickly move the leg and then apply enough strength to prevent the body from tipping over.

Vestibular System

Although the vestibular system is composed of several subsystems as mentioned above, the principal vestibular system is associated

Table 2–1. The Three Components of the Balance System

Vestibular	Visual	Somatosensory
Inner ear (labrynthine)	Eyes (vision)	Sensors in legs, muscles, and joints

with the inner ear structures, namely, the **semicircular canals**, the **utricle**, and **saccule** (Figure 2-1). Sensory "hair" cells found within these structures are similar to those found in the hearing organ (cochlea) but respond to the movement of surrounding fluids instead of sound. The semicircular canals respond to angular acceleration of the head turning in any direction.

As seen in Figure 2-1, each semicircular canal is oriented in a different plane, allowing for sensation of movement of the head in the forward-backward direction ("posterior" canal), back and forth direction ("horizontal" canal), or tipping side to side ("anterior" canal). Canals are situated slightly off center to allow for detection of movements that are not exactly in these planes. In addition to the semicircular canals, the utricle and saccule contain hair cells that are situated to detect linear motion. Specifically, the saccule detects movement mainly in the "up" or "down" direction such as when riding in an elevator; whereas the utricle detects movement in the horizontal plane, such as "forward" or "backward" directions, as may be felt, for example, when accelerating forward in a car. The hair cell structures themselves are somewhat different in the semicircular canals than in the utricle or saccule. In the semicircular canals, the hair cells are housed within the crista ampullaris, a structure found within a bulging area at the end of each semicircular canal referred to as the **ampulla**. Hairs are embedded within a gelatinous membrane above, called the **cupula**. The utricle and saccule however, have an additional component, the "**otoliths**." The term otolith refers to calcium carbonate crystals, sometimes called "ear rocks" (*oto* = ear; *lyth* = rock) that are embedded in the gelatinous layer above the hairs. These crystals give added weight to the gelatinous layer allowing it to pull more forcefully on the hairs in response to fluid movement. The disadvantage of the otoliths is that some of these may break free and fall to areas where they do not belong, primarily into the ampullae or semicircular canals. This condition is thought to result in "benign positional vertigo," one of the conditions in which head movements cause a severe spinning sensation ("vertigo"). Movement-caused vertigo is usually due to a vestibular disorder, but can occasionally be caused by central nervous system (CNS) problems. More on positional vertigo and movement-related vertigo is covered in a later section of this chapter.

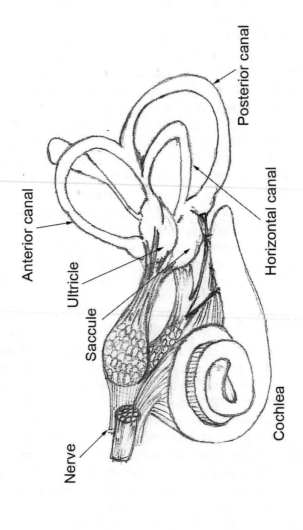

Figure 2–1. The vestibular system showing orientation of the semicircular canals.

Figure 2-2 shows a detailed view of the hair cell structures, the cupula, and cristae. Fluid surrounding the hair cell structures is endolymph, which is continuous with the endolymph of the cochlea.

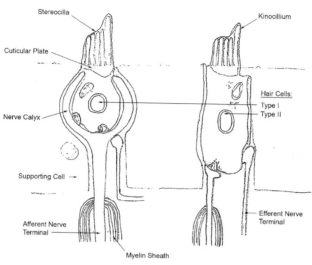

A.

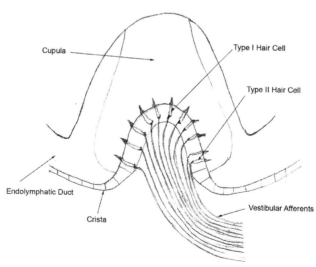

B.

Figure 2–2. **A.** Type I and type II hair cell structure. **B.** Hair cells within the cupula.

The "Ear–Eye Connection"

The **vestibular-ocular reflex** or **VOR** refers to the interconnections between the ear balance organs just described and the muscles of the eyes. These interconnections also explain why the eyes sometimes jerk involuntarily ("**nystagmus**") when there is an inner-ear balance system disorder. More about nystagmus is explained in the section below.

The VOR, shown diagrammatically in Figure 2–3, causes the eyes to move in the opposite direction of the head, thus allowing a visual image to remain on the retina. For example, a head movement to the right, which mainly stimulates the **horizontal semicircular canals**, results in a rapid reflexive eye movement in the opposite direction (left). As shown in Figure 2–3, this eye move-

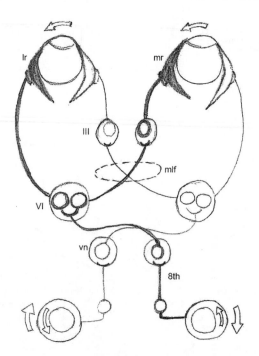

Figure 2–3. The vestibulo-ocular reflex pathway (VOR). In this example, for a head turn to the right, the right ear horizontal canal is excitatory and moves the eyes to the left.

ment is explained by the innervation pathways that cross to the opposite side within the brainstem. The fluid in the right horizontal canal moves relatively toward the right ear's horizontal canal ampulla (ampullopedal movement), causing an increased firing rate of the nerve on the right side. This causes an increased response to the left eye's lateral rectus muscle and the right eye's medial rectus muscle causing them to contract pulling the eye to the left. At the same time this is happening, there is a decreased response of the opposing muscles caused by ampullofugal fluid movement (away from the ampulla) in the left ear, which causes a decreased firing rate further allowing the eye to move easily leftward (assuming the patient is in the dark and not fixating on a visual target). After this pulling of the eye to the left (the vestibular phase), the CNS quickly pulls the eye back to the right. Similar eye movements for other directions are produced by responses of the other semicircular canals to movement in their respective planes. The VOR can also be continuously stimulated by disease in that ear or caloric irrigation, creating a repetitive back and forth movement of the eyes, **nystagmus**. This may occur if there is an irritative lesion or warm irrigation on the right side as in an ENG/VNG examination. Similarly, nystagmus could be created by accelerating the patient in a rightward direction such as in a rotational chair test, or if the head is thrust quickly to the right as in a manual head thrust test.

The manner in which head movement affects eye movement by way of the VOR can be explained by the following example. As shown in Figure 2–3, movement of the head to the right causes the fluid in the horizontal canal to move to the left relative to the canal. This movement of fluid toward the ampulla (in this case of the right ear) results in a slow eye movement to the left and rapid return to the right.

Nystagmus

The mechanism of the VOR just explained, also helps to explain **nystamgus**. Nystagmus, which is involuntary eye jerking, is usually abnormal and may be due to either an inner ear or central nervous system disorder. Nystagmus may also be "artificially" created by rapid continuous acceleration or caloric irrigation. When nystagmus is due to an abnormal inner ear usually only one ear is producing the problem. This can be illustrated by a caloric irrigation to one ear using cool or warm air or water. For example, if only the right ear is stimulated for several seconds by warm water, the same pulling of the eyes to the left as described above would occur due to stimulation of the right inner ear mechanism. If in the dark or with eyes closed, the eyes do not remain to the left, but are quickly brought back to the original position by the central nervous system. This latter movement is much quicker than the first; thus, the vestibular component of the nystagmus is the slow component, whereas the fast component represents the central component. Nystagmus is labeled by its fast component; therefore, the nystagmus produced in this example is "right beating," which is toward the side of warm irrigation. Cool irrigation of the same ear, however, decreases neural firing and results in an opposite beating nystagmus direction. The mnemonic "COWS ("Cold Opposite, Warm Same") refers to this direction relationship. Actual ear disorders may be either **ablative** such as in those caused by a tumor, severed nerve, or cool water irrigation. Less frequently, an **irritative lesion** may occur such as in certain phases of Ménière's disease or from a warm irrigation. Nystagmus is also caused in normals by rotating the patient in the dark such as during rotational chair testing. Nystagmus occurs with the fast phase in the direction of rotation; however, as the labrynthine system is sensitive mainly to acceleration, nystagmus will occur mainly during periods of acceleration or deceleration such as at the beginning or end of a continuous speed rotation.

Nystagmus may also have a nonotologic etiology (CNS) in which case it usually takes on different forms. Nystagmus that is caused by the peripheral vestibular system has certain identifiable characteristics. Table 2–2 shows the differences in characteristics of peripheral versus central nystagmus that *usually* occur. As shown in Table 2–2, peripheral nystagmus is usually worse in the dark or behind closed eyelids, beats away from the offending ear (assuming an ablative disorder as explained above), is suppressed or absent with eyes open fixating on a target, and is enhanced when gazing in the direction of the fast phase (Alexander's law). The last characteristic is not always observable because the eyes are open and fixating. This problem can usually be overcome by the use of video goggles with eyes covered or by using electro-oculography (ENG)

Table 2–2. Nystagmus Characteristics

Peripheral Vestibular	Central Vestibular or Other Central Nystagmus
Greater or only present with vision denied	Greater with eyes open, or the same with eyes open or closed
Enhanced when gaze in direction of fast phase (Alexander's law)	Present only on side gaze with eyes open

electrodes at the sides of the eyes with eyes closed. Peripheral nystagmus is seldom beating up or down due presumably to the dominance of the horizontal semicircular canal system over the anterior or posterior. In contrast, central nystagmus may mimic peripheral nystagmus in some cases; however, it typically lacks some of the characteristics of peripheral nystagmus. Central nystagmus may beat down or up, may be worse with eyes open, only present with eyes open, or the same with eyes open or closed. It may be disrhythmic, or exihibit other unusual characteristics. In addition, central nystagmus may only be present during gaze. This latter characteristic, however, may confuse it with peripheral nystagmus that, if very mild, may only be discernible during the gaze enhancement, noted just above, behind closed video goggles. Gaze nystagmus may also be produced in normals when gazing greater than 30 degrees off center. This nystagmus, which would have its fast phase in the direction of the gaze, is termed **endpoint nystagmus** and is usually only present in the dark or with eyes covered. When examining the patient without equipment, significant nystagmus that is present only with eyes open either signifies a central lesion or the patient is in the middle of an acute vestibular attack.

Rotational or Torsional Nystagmus

Also called rotational nystagmus, torsional nystagmus is common and usually a sign of peripheral vestibular disorder, specifically, **benign paroxysmal positional vertigo (BPPV)**; however, rotational nystagmus may also have central etiology. This nystagmus is covered in more detail later in this chapter in the section on benign paroxysmal positional vertigo (BPPV).

Other Vestibular Subsystems

Besides the VOR, there are other vestibular subsystems, including the vestibulospinal tracts, vestibular-cerebellar interactions, cervicovestibular system, and others. All of these are coordinated within the brainstem, mostly within the vestibular nuclei in the **pons**. The vestibulospinal tract represents connections between the vestibular nuclei and the extremities. This system is demonstrated when the arm or leg of the opposite side extends reflexively if the body suddenly tilts off center. The cervicovestibular system consists of connections between the vestibular system and neck receptors found in the deep regions of the vertebrae. This system is demonstrated in an animal model. While holding a rabbit upright, keeping the rabbit's head in a constant upright position, the neck is stressed by tilting the rabbit's body either right or left. The rabbit's eyes will move to the opposite side of body movement. Of these various subsystems, the vestibulospinal tracts are the best understood and appreciated. Physical therapists also recognize the importance of the neck and back to proper balance function.

Common Vestibular Disorders

Common "vestibular" ("ear") disorders causing vertigo of varying degree as well as mild imbalance include **benign paroxysmal positional vertigo (BPPV)**, **vestibular neuronitis**, **viral labrynthitis**, **sudden sensorineural hearing loss**, **Ménière's disease**, **acoustic schwanoma**, **perilymphatic fistula**, **superior canal dehiscence**, as well as **central vestibular** disorders due to pathologies in the brainstem or cerebellum. The vestibular system technically also includes areas of the cortex, abnormalities of which can also cause symptoms of vertigo or imbalance.

In summary, the vestibular system is complex and consists of several subsystems. The inner-ear or labrynthine vestibular system is well understood, and is often the cause of abnormal balance ranging from cases of severe dizziness to mild or position-induced imbalance.

Visual Balance System

Notwithstanding the large number of balance complaints caused by vestibular disorder, the vestibular system still is considered the least important of the balance systems. Consider, for example, that the deaf frequently lose this system entirely when contracting the deafness. For one or two months, the patient is extremely dizzy, but in the end, this disability is largely compensated for by the visual and somatosensory systems. If this were not true, many or most deaf individuals would be off balance most of the time. This, however, is obviously not the case, which demonstrates that the visual and somatosensory balance systems do an impressive job of compensating. It is true that the deaf who have affected vestibular systems often have reduced sensitivity for balance when in darkened environments and often use a wider based gait than is typical. The eye balance system, therefore, is recognized as being more important on a basic level than the vestibular (ear) balance system. It is amazing how accurate the eye's system for judging the horizontal is, being able, for example, to tell a picture that is not straight within a fraction of an inch. This visual system, of course, is reduced in effectiveness in environments where light is not adequate. Surprisingly though, the sense of vision is useful even when only the memory of what we have seen in the past is being used. We have all had the experience of navigating a darkened room successfully based on our visual memory of what the room was like when it was lighter.

Somatosensory Balance System

Also high on the list of important balance systems is the somatosensory system, by which we sense the position of portions of our body, legs, and feet using the nerves (proprioceptors) found within the joints and muscles. This is the system by which we can tell how high our foot is being raised without looking at it. This ability is a learned behavior and requires some time after birth before we can sense the location of our body in relation to the ground by using only the feeling in our extremities. Abnormalities of the somatosensory balance system make it difficult for persons to walk well on uneven or soft surfaces. Such is also the case, however, with vestibular disorders.

Gait and Mobility

Normal gait and mobility require adequate **nervous system function**, termed **"sensory and motor function,"** adequate **"structural" features** of the lower extremities, and normal **muscular function**. An example of nervous system disorder is Parkinson's disease, in which the basal ganglia of the brain do not integrate normally with the motor cortex allowing for normal neural messages to be sent to the legs. Examples of abnormal "structural features" affecting mobility are deformity of the limbs or simple joint stiffness due to arthritis, which itself can result in abnormal movements. Another example of "abnormal" structure causing abnormal movement is obesity. As obese persons have 10% higher "net metabolic rate" for normal walking than persons of normal weight, it takes more energy for an obese person to walk (Browning et al., 2006); therefore, gait and stamina are sometimes affected. An example of a muscular disorder affecting movement is myasthenia gravis, which can disallow adequate muscle function for the movements necessary for normal walking.

Among the many mobility affecting disorders are stroke, multiple sclerosis, Parkinson's disease, traumatic brain injuries, spinal disorders or injuries, congenital abnormalities, obesity, arthritis, and balance disorders.

Gait

Normal gait requires a complex combination of functions involving neural, muscular, and related functions. Physicians know from experience that much can be determined about a person's overall health simply by observing the patient's gait. Even specific diagnoses can be made based upon a person's gait. Normal gait is a complex function in which approximately 25 separate muscles are involved in normal movement of the lower extremities while walking. Gait has been analyzed for various reasons and under varying degrees of technical sophistication. For example, in a very technical analysis, Ayyappa (1997) divided gait into several phases, such as "initial contact," "initial swing," "midswing," and "terminal swing," each having characteristic leg and foot positions. Such complex analyses are greater than needed for clinical assessment. The goal for most clinicians working with fall-prone individuals should not be to make specific diagnoses based on gait, but rather to be able to recognize when gait is abnormal and how the abnormality may be contributing to falls. It is also important to distinguish between abnormal gait due to pathology and abnormal gait due to "normal" aging. This comes with experience. Recognizing a few common abnormal gait types that are suggestive of common disorders is a useful skill for the effective clinician. Through assessment of a patient's gait, the clinician can more effectively plan falls-prevention strategies.

A great deal of information is available concerning gait and balance in both normals and abnormals. A wide variety of disciplines are interested in this subject both from the standpoint of diagnosis as well as rehabilitation. Disciplines having particular interest in this subject are neurology, rehabilitation medicine, podiatry, exercise physiology, physical therapy, as well as primary caregivers. The field of "biomechanics" in particular studies gait and motion in the laboratory.

Both abnormal gait and abnormal mobility have been shown to be independently associated with increased falls (Liu-Ambrose et al., 2006). Abnormally slow gait has been associated with increased falls and the assessment of gait speed has promise as an individual test for predicting falls (Montero-Odasso et al., 2005).

Recognizing Normal Gait

Many textbooks and papers dealing with gait do not describe normal gait as much as they do abnormal gait. This is partly because gait is highly variable among normal individuals making it difficult to recognize abnormal gait. However, becoming familiar with normal gait is important because then we can recognize abnormal gait more effectively, even when it is not certain what the abnormality is. The uninitiated observer will first think that most patients have abnormal gait. This is partly because everyone walks somewhat differently; however, it should be realized that gait does not have to be "pretty" to be normal. Persons with normal gait often look abnormal because, when observing the body as a whole, there are many divergent or unusual body sizes and shapes which may give the person an unusual effect while walking. The evaluation of gait is therefore a somewhat subjective endeavor and the clinician should evaluate gait with consideration of such issues as "ease of walking," "speed according to body size," and especially "general stability." The question in the examiner's mind should be, "why is this person's gait abnormal?" Is the abnormality due to mostly intrinsic medical factors, or could the abnormality be due to more mundane or simpler issues such as ingrown toenails, extremes in footwear, use of bifocals when looking down, or impracticality of the person's walking device or cane. Abnormal gait is not only caused by neurologic or muscular disorders but can be caused by more common leg abnormalities, with arthritis and peripheral vascular disease being two of the most common (Hinman et al., 2002). Even when the cause of abnormal gait is intrinsic, the issue can be entirely unrelated to the lower extremities such as in poor vision or obesity. In the latter case, the obesity may not always affect gait if there is adequate muscle strength and conditioning sufficient to control the gait. In obesity, a person's trunk may lean, or the arms may not hang straight down; therefore, the weight of the person's upper body may cause the trunk to tilt forward or some other unnatural direction.

Evidence is also beginning to emerge that gait disorders may be due solely to dementia, independent of any other neurologic deficit or dysfunction of the muscles or limbs themselves. In one study by Salazar, Vandenberg, and Potter (2002), gait disorders were present even in many having mild dementia. Gait disorders tend to also be present in those with Alzheimer's disease.

In short, the ability to make effective analysis of gait is based on experience which increases over time; nevertheless, learning some fundamentals about normal gait is a good first step. Despite the variability mentioned above in normals, there are certain elements of normal walking that are present in most normals. A useful description of normal gait has been provided by Tinetti (1986). In the section below, "Elements of Normal Gait," we provide our interpretation of most of the major aspects of the Tinetti criteria for normal gait. Suggestions on how to best observe a patient's gait have also been offered by Blumenfeld (2002). Accordingly, the patient should be observed walking both toward and away from the examiner. The gait examination should include detailed notes that may compare the patient's gait from one visit to the next. We have also found it important to observe the patient walking at least the distance of 100 feet with a visual target ahead. Distances that somewhat tax the individual offer the advantage of being able to observe the patient when slightly fatigued as might actually occur during a longer walk. Gait may significantly deteriorate with distance. It is important to have the patient wear a safety harness or physical therapy belt around the waist to prevent any falls during gait testing. During the analysis, the patient should be given the opportunity to make a turn in either direction.

Elements of Normal Gait

Initiation of gait: The patient can initiate gait immediately in a single smooth motion without hesitation. The initiation of gait seems natural and almost effortless.

Feet clear the floor: The swinging foot completely clears the floor; however, it still comes quite close to touching the floor.

Step distance: The distance between the heel of the forward foot and the toe of the following foot should be about the length of the person's foot and is usually a bit longer. In aging individuals, step length becomes somewhat smaller. The step length should be about the same on both sides.

Smooth and continuous: The heel of the back foot begins to rise at about the time the heel of front foot touches the floor. There are no stops or breaks in stride and the step length is equal over most cycles.

Deviation: The person walks in a fairly straight line.

Trunk stability: The arms are to the side as they swing and the trunk does not sway. The knees or back are not flexed.

Stance: When observing from behind, the patient's feet almost touch as one passes the other.

Turning: When turning, steps are continuous. There is no staggering.

Changes in Gait with Aging

Through experience, the examiner should eventually be able to differentiate "normal" changes in gait due to aging from abnormal gait caused by disease states that need further assessment. Some normal aging adults have fairly normal gait well into advanced age. It is more typical, however, for the aging individual to have smaller steps (reduced length of stride) and reduced velocity of gait. Changes in gait with normal aging are described in the *Merck Manual of Geriatrics 2000-2006* (Beers, Jones, Berkwitz, Kaplan, & Porter, 2006), as summarized below:

> **Velocity:** Walking generally slows, starting at about age 70. Velocity is slower more because steps are shorter rather than the speed of steps being less.
>
> **Cadence (frequency or rhythm of walking):** Does not change much with age. Speed of steps (cadence) depends more on body size and shape, with taller people taking longer but slower steps, and shorter people taking shorter steps at a faster cadence.
>
> **Double stance:** This is the amount of time both feet are on the ground together during walking. Usually, this occurs for only a very short amount of time, but in older individuals this time increases because the body is more stable if both feet are supporting the body at the same time.
>
> **Greater "toe out" foot position:** Older individuals walk with the feet pointed slightly more laterally (outward). This is only a slight change from when younger (about 5 degrees).
>
> **Smaller steps:** Possibly due to reduced strength in calf muscles. This also may be due to the person being more wary of falls, and therefore more reluctant to take longer steps as this would decrease the amount of time in "double stance" (see above), thus causing more time that there is only one foot on the ground for support.

There are also some additional minor changes in gait with age, but these may be too minor to observe easily. For example, there are slight changes in joint motion during walking in the aging individual.

Although many of the changes in gait with aging may be considered "normal," such changes are nonetheless often detrimental to ambulation and can lead to situations that can cause falls. For example, the smaller step lengths and slower speed naturally cause the person to take longer to get somewhere. On the other hand, the slower speed and smaller steps are a natural way for the person to avoid falling because of the instability that may occur at higher speeds. However, being slower and using smaller steps can lead to increased falls in situations where more speed is necessary such as when crossing a street at a crossing signal. In our clinic, a common cause of falling is rushing to answer the telephone or the doorbell.

Describing Abnormal Gait

A convenient way of describing abnormal gait is to use the terminology of Tinetti or Beers in the sections above, describing the patient's gait as having abnormal "deviation," "step distance," and so forth. A general summary statement of the patient's gait in terms of its potential to cause falls is also appropriate. Examples: "Overall, the patient's gait is very unstable with incidents of near falls," "The patient's occasional dragging of a toe presents significant risk for falls," and so forth. This ties the gait description to what it may mean to the patient in terms of falls.

Other Common Descriptors of Abnormal Gait

Just as observations of gait require some subjectivity, it is also acceptable that descriptions of gait include some subjective wording in order to be more descriptive and give the reader a visual picture of the patient's gait. Descriptive wording is necessary due to the wide variety of deviant gait patterns. Words such as "staggering," "near falling," and "halting" are useful in giving the reader a visualization of the patient's gait and ambulation problems. Despite these appropriate subjective descriptions, there is a certain amount of standard terminology applied to abnormal gait. Many of these terms have been described by Blumenfeld (2002). The following is our interpretation of many of these:

> **Spastic gait:** Spastic pattern, circumduction or stiff-legged, example, MS.

> **Ataxic gait:** A broad term meaning any of the following—wide-based, staggering, unsteady, falling (may be subtle and detected only with more difficult

task such as tandem gait); example, cerebellar abnormality.

Vertiginous gait (vestibular gait): Similar to ataxic gait, but worse with movement of head. Example, vestibular neuritis may result in a lingering uncompensated vestibulopathy causing the gait to be worse when walking while moving the head.

Frontal (lobe) gait: A characteristic shuffling, slow, wide or narrow based gait, barely raising feet, resembles Parkinsonian gait, but some can do cycling movements with legs while lying on their back but not on their feet (this causes some to use the term "apraxic gait." Example, diffuse subcortical white matter disease may cause this type of gait.

Parkinsonian gait: Characteristic difficulty initiating gait, narrow based but slow, shuffling; example, Parkinson's disease.

Functional: Gait problems are inconsistent. For example, at times, can perform difficult movements unexpectedly to the observer.

Antalgic gait: Abnormal gait due to pain, such as a limp due to pain. Other examples include herniated disk, peripheral neuropathy, fracture, arthritis with pain in ankles or knees.

Tabetic gait: High steps, foot flopping, difficulty on uneven surfaces; example, posterior cord or severe sensory neuropathy.

Orthopedic gait disorder: Abnormal gait due to injury or disorder of a limb or may sometimes be due to spinal cord deficit.

Paretic gait: Variable, can be tripping, knee buckling, high stepping with foot drop, waddling, Trendelenberg gait; example, muscle or peripheral nerves.

Dyskinetic gait: Flinging, dancelike, or writhing; example, Huntington's disease.

Common Causes of Abnormal Gait in the Falls Clinic

Individuals with a wide variety of disorders causing abnormal gait present to the falls clinic. Most serious disorders have often been diagnosed prior to presenting to the clinic such as neurologic, spinal cord problems, degenerative muscular disorders. and others. Although a patient may have been diagnosed long ago with a serious disorder such as Parkinson's disease, what is often lacking on arrival at the clinic is an appreciation of the problems in gait and potential falling that such a disorder may be causing the individual. Determining these effects on balance and falls can only be appreciated by direct observation of the gait and is one of the primary purposes of examining gait and balance in the falls clinic. Although most patients with medical disorders causing abnormal gait arrive in the falls clinic having been previously diagnosed, some disorders affecting gait will first be discovered in the falls or balance clinic. Although vestibular disorders are very common, more common disorders such as arthritis of the knees or ankles often are found to be the primary cause of falls. An example is foot pain, which can be caused by a variety of disorders. Simply the pain itself can cause abnormal gait and, therefore, contribute to falls. Determining the true cause of falls is largely based on observation of the patient under various walking situations or during the informal balance assessment described in Chapter 5. The following brief example is instructive.

Example Case

A 75-year-old male presents to the clinic with complaints of imbalance whenever walking but never has dizziness while sitting or lying. Vestibular testing shows mild bilateral vestibular weakness. The patient exhibits a markedly abnormal ataxic gait, characterized by moderate staggering and near falling at times. On examination of the lower extremities, it is noted that the patient has weakness in the knees bilaterally and pain in the knees due to arthritis. A chart review also shows a previous diagnosis of cerebellar degeneration, consistent with the apraxic gait.

   This case demonstrates the common dilemma of a patient presenting with two or more abnormalities that can be affecting the gait, in this case the vestibulopathy, cerebellar degeneration, and the arthritic problems. During the practical examination of the patient's gait and balance, it was obvious that the bulk of this patient's problem with falling lies in the lack of normal leg function. This determination is made by observing the patient's gait, as well as performance on a combination of practical balance tasks. It is noted that the patient can stand on foam for several seconds with the eyes closed, demonstrating that the vestibular problem is not causing major balance problems, at least when the patient is standing still (static balance). Observing the gait, there is marked staggering and near falling. The patient fails a simple coordination test of the lower extremities (running the heel of one foot down the length of the other leg from the knee to the ankle). As to the arthritis, simply questioning the patient was enlightening. The patient was able to perceive that the pain was not contributing to any difference in his walking ability because the pain is only intermittent. Therefore, the patient was able to compare his walking with and without pain, determining that there is no significant difference. These combined results, especially simply observing the patient while walking, lead to the conclusion that, although the patient does have mild bilateral vestibular weakness, the nature of his problem in a practical sense was due more to his inability to move his legs properly. Although it is true that the mildly decreased sense of vestibular balance added to the patient's difficulties, particularly in darkened environments, the greatest problem causing falls likely was the patient's leg challenges. With this combined information, strategies for falls prevention are now more easily prioritized, in this case, therapy would emphasize the leg problems.

Summary

In summary, adequate balance and mobility are prerequisites to standing or walking without falls. Abnormality in any of the balance and gait functions described in this chapter can easily lead to falls. Assessment of the three components of the balance system, visual, somatosensory, and vestibular as well as gait and mobility function is critical to determining the cause of falls.

Balance Disorders

Vestibular Disorders

Vestibular disorders usually refer to the "inner ear" balance system and related mechanisms. Vertigo usually is the symptom that distinguishes a vestibular disorder, although vertigo can occasionally be present in cerebral disorders. **Vertigo** is the term employed to indicate a true hallucination of motion or spinning sensation, whereas the term "**dizziness**," described fully in Chapter 4, is more general and is not always used consistently by patients. What is sometimes confusing, however, is the fact that in many cases of vestibular disorder, the vertigo can often be a mild, even vague sensation. Although there is sometimes frank spinning, more often terms such as "floating" or "woozy" are used by the patient when describing the vertigo. Although we do not have to rely on symptoms alone to differentiate between vestibular and nonvestibular disorders; nevertheless, the history is critical in determining vestibular disorders. Symptoms usually include "being a little off," particularly made worse with "quick movements," "worse in the dark," or "worse with head or body position changes" particularly bending down, looking up or turning from side to side in bed. These symptoms are due to the fact that the inner ear mechanism is naturally responsive to movement.

In vestibular disorder, our sense of body position or motion may be either reduced (hypoactive) or abnormally enhanced (hyperactive). In the hypoactive case, we could turn while walking in the dark (without vision) and not be aware that a turn has occurred. In such a case, we would have a reduced sensation of motion. In contrast, in the hyperactive case, the slightest turn may make us feel as if we are spinning. These two symptoms, hyperactive or hypoactive response to movement, can be created by a variety of vestibular disorders, some of which could cause either symptom.

Nystagmus, assuming that it is the "peripheral type," is the hallmark sign of a vestibular disorder. However, because visual fixation inhibits peripheral nystagmus, it is usually seen clinically only in the dark, that is, behind closed video goggles or while using Frenzel's lenses to disallow visual fixation. Therefore, assuming that the patient has not just moved the head rapidly, if nystagmus is seen at center gaze with eyes open in a lighted room, the patient either has a CNS disorder or is in the most acute stages of a peripheral vestibular disorder (within a week or so of its onset). Vestibular nystagmus is, therefore, often missed in routine clinical examinations without equipment that allows the eyes to be visualized in the dark. Earlier in this chapter, we discussed the difference between vestibular- and CNS-caused nystagmus (see earlier sections). Testing and screening methods for nystagmus and vestibular disorders are outlined in greater detail in Chapter 5.

Common Disorders

BPPV (Benign Paroxysmal Positional Vertigo)

One of the most common disorders, **benign paroxysmal positional vertigo or BPPV**, is distinguished by a positive Hallpike (Nylen-Barany) test; however, may not be determined easily by symptoms alone. The classic symptoms of "dizzy when looking up or bending over" or "dizzy when I first rise from bed or first lie down" are frequently not given. A vague complaint of "mild dizziness," "a little off," or "woozy" is often given instead. Such patients with vague histories will still often show an abnormal Hallpike test. On the other hand, a positive Hallpike is not always present in patients with BPPV, or may only be present at certain times. It is wise to retest the Hallpike more than once in these patients, as it is the author's experience that the Hallpike may be present only during the second or third trial, even when performed on the same day. Fortunately, "canalith repositioning maneuvers" are currently successful in alleviating BPPV symptoms in most people. It should be noted that BPPV is often not an isolated otologic disorder, but is found in combination with other more serious ear disorders. A positive Hallpike infrequently may also be seen in CNS disorders, although the test is usually "atypical" in these cases in that the response may not fatigue or have other unusual signs.

Bilateral Weakness (Reduced Vestibular Response Bilaterally)

To some extent, older individuals frequently lose their fine ability to sense motion. Similar to the loss of hearing due to aging, there is often a reduction in the vestibular response. Such a balance problem can occur separately from a hearing problem or in conjunction with one. Although the inner ear houses both the hearing and balance mechanisms, these are found in separate areas although they share some common fluids (endolymph and perilymph (see Figure 2-2). Because the two mechanisms are separate, hearing loss can occur without a balance problem and vice versa. On the other hand, because of the close proximity of these two mechanisms some disorders can affect both hearing and balance.

A bilateral reduced vestibular response may also be due to a past toxicity of the balance mechanism by medication. This ototoxicity (or vestibulotoxicity as it is sometimes called) is even more likely when kidney disease is present. In many cases, however, bilateral reduced vestibular response is due to unknown causes and possibly due to aging alone. Just as the term "presbycusis" refers to loss of hearing due to aging, the term "presbystasis" has been suggested to refer to the condition of losing inner ear balance due to gradual aging.

Other common vestibular disorders include vestibular neuritis, ototoxicity, and nonspecific uncompensated vestibulopathy. Less common are perilymphatic fistula, superior canal dehiscence, viral labrynthitis, Ménière's syndrome, acoustic schwanoma, and sudden sensorineural hearing loss with dizziness. Disorders sometimes confused with vestibulopathy from a patient history standpoint include postural hypotension, migraine complex, brain tumor, psychogenic disorder, hyperventilation, ocular disorders, cardiovascular disorder, and neurologic causes.

Somatosensory Disorders

Problems with a sense of body position can also occur in **somatosensory/proprioceptive** disturbances. The somatosensory system refers to nerves that allow the ability to consciously sense pain, touch, temperature, or vibration. Proprioceptors are nerve receptors in the limbs or joints that allow the sense of position of a limb. These important systems help to determine the body's position and respond as needed. It should be noted that portions of the vestibular system also are involved in muscle responses to position changes, such as the vestibulospinal tract, which sends motor signals to the arms and legs as well as other areas. The way in which the vestibular and somatosensory systems work simultaneously can be shown by the following example. If we step onto a slanted surface in the dark, both the somatosensory and vestibular systems may sense that we are now standing on a tilted surface. The vestibular system, by way of the vestibulospinal tract, would send motor signals to extend an arm or leg to help counterbalance our tipping. In addition, the somatosensory system would "feel" the slant, which would then signal an appropriate muscle to react in order to stabilize balance. Although the vestibular and visual systems are extremely important, the importance of the muscle balance systems can be appreciated when one considers that persons without either the vestibular system (some deaf individuals) or the visual system (the blind) can do quite well with balance without having one or both of these systems. This fact emphasizes the potential for rehabilitation in persons lacking function in any of the three balance systems.

Visual Disorders

Visual perceptions of the body's surroundings form an important component of balance. Visual disorders possibly affecting balance include abnormal visual acuity, depth perception, contrast vision, or eye movement. Central nervous system disorders affecting balance, such as multiple sclerosis, can also adversely affect visual balance.

Vestibular nystagmus is not usually considered an "eye disorder" but nevertheless forms the basis of the vertigo and imbalance experienced in vestibular disorders. It should be remembered that nystagmus can also occasionally occur in CNS disorders.

Another abnormal eye movement, oscillopsia, is usually caused by peripheral vestibular disorder. Oscillopsia refers to the eye movements occurring abnormally in response to body movement, due to the inability of the vestibular ocular reflex to maintain the visual image on the fovea of the retina. For example, there may be a bouncing of the eyes in response to walking, causing the visual image also to bounce. In extreme cases, the patient may complain that it is difficult to read signs while walking because the words jump around or jiggle. More commonly, the eye movement is less obvious to the patient or examiner and is often difficult to see without using video goggles after head shaking (vision denied), in which case an actual nystagmus would be seen.

Other abnormal eye movements include "oculomotor" abnormalities such as the inability to follow a smoothly moving target (smooth pursuit or pendular tracking), producing a jerky "cogwheeling" pattern or complete inability to follow the target, abnormal rapid eye movement control (as in the saccade test), or "disconjugate" eye movements, in which the eyes do not move together smoothly at all times. The latter disorder can sometimes be seen easier without equipment and may look normal on VNG or ENG unless a separate recording channel is used for each eye.

Neurologic Disorders

Brain and other neurologic disorders can cause more bizarre forms of spatial hallucination, with or without a sense of motion, which can also result in falls. Major disease in nearly any part of the brain is theoretically capable of causing a distorted perception of our surroundings. There is hardly a major area of the brain (lobe) that does not participate in assessing our surroundings visually or tactilely. The parietal lobe is particularly involved in spatial orientation; the occipital and frontal lobes are involved in vision and eye movement; and the temporal and parietal lobes have been implicated in the perceptions of vertigo.

Neurologic disorders can impair balance and cause falls in a variety of ways by affecting sensation, perception, or movement function. Ability to move normally may be affected in **movement disorders** such as Parkinson's disease. **Perceptual disturbances** of surroundings or self also are possible in neurologic disorders. Reduced sensation in the lower extremities is often caused by peripheral neuropathy, but can also be due to central nervous system involvements such as in lumbar spine disorders. **Neuromuscular** disorders may also affect a person's strength or ability to stand or walk. However, if the loss of strength is throughout the body, then **generalized body weakness** is usually the cause and most often is due to metabolic, muscular, or cardiogenic disorders.

References

Ayyappa, E. (1997). Normal human locomotion: Part 1. Basic concepts and terminology. *Journal of Prosthetics and Orthotics, 9*(1), 10-17.

Beers, M, H., Jones, T. V., Berkwits, M., Kaplan, J. L., & Porter, R. (Eds.). (2006). *The Merck manual of geriatrics* (3rd ed., Updated, 2000-2006). Whitehouse Station, NY: Merck and Co. (http://www.merck.com/mrkshared/mmg/home.jsp).

Blumenfeld, H. (2002). The neurologic exam as a lesson in neuroanatomy. In *Neuroanatomy through clinical cases* (p. 70). Sunderland, MA: Sinauer Associates.

Browning, R. C., Baker, E. A;, Herron, J. A., & Kram, R. (2006). Effects of obesity and sex on the energetic cost and preferred speed of walking. *Journal of Applied Physiology, 100*(2), 390-398.

Gardner, A. W. (2001). Altered gait profile in subjects with peripheral arterial disease. *Vascular Medicine, 6*(1), 31-34.

Hinman, R. S., Bennell, K. L., Metcalf, B. R., & Crossley, K. M. (2002). Balance impairments in individuals with symptomatic knee osteoarthritis: A comparison with matched controls using clinical tests. *Rheumatology, 41*, 1388-1394.

Liu-Ambrose, T., Khan, K. M., Donaldson, M. G., Eng, J. J., Lord, S. R., & McKay, H. A. (2006). Falls-related self-efficacy is independently associated with balance and mobility in older women with low bone mass. *Journals of Gerontology Series A: Biological Sciences and Medical Sciences, 61*, 832-838.

Montero-Odasso, M., Schapira, M., Soriano, E. R., Varela, M., Kaplan, R., Camera, L. A., & Mayorga, L. M. (2005). Gait velocity as a single predictor of adverse events in healthy seniors aged 75 years and older. *Journals of Gerontology Series A: Biological Sciences and Medical Sciences, 60*, 1304-1309.

Salazar, T. V., Vandenberg, E. V., & Potter, J. F. (2002). Non-neurological factors are implicated in impairments in gait and mobility among patients in a clinical dementia referral population. *International Journal of Geriatric Psychiatry, 17*(2), 128-133.

Tinetti, M. E. (1986). Performance-oriented assessment of mobility problems in elderly patients. *Journal of the American Geriatrics Society, 34*, 119-126.

CHAPTER 3

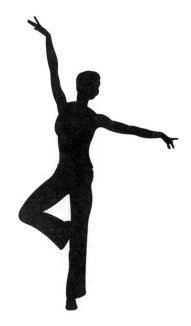

Why We Fall

Falls Theory

We all can relate to the experience of falling. Although we may not remember falling as toddlers, most of us can remember falling many times as children and, hopefully, only occasionally as adults. With a little reflection we realize that maintaining balance on two feet is a complex task; therefore, it is easy to realize that there are a multitude of causes of falls.

Much has been written on the topic of falls. Most of the focus in the literature deals with "risk factors," which means the medical conditions or other "extrinsic" factors that lead to falls. We will take a fresh start on the topic from a theoretical standpoint.

Excepting catastrophic events, **there are only two possible reasons we fall**:

1. **We do not sense or realize that we are tipping, or**
2. **We cannot stop ourselves while tipping.**

Although these reasons seem obvious, there are many factors relating to each of these two basic reasons for falling. The first of these reasons, **not realizing we are tipping**, is due to either a loss of sensory information to the brain or a loss of awareness of that information. We may not "sense" that we are falling because of a deficit in one or more of the three **sensory balance systems** discussed in Chapter 2, **somatosensory** (sometimes termed the "leg" balance system although other parts of the body are also involved), **visual balance system**, or **vestibular system** (inner ear and associated neural connections). An example of not realizing we are tipping is given by the following scenario. Imagine a person having an inner-ear balance system disturbance (vestibular disorder) walking down the isle of a dark theater. Without the visual input, this person relies more on the vestibular (inner ear) balance system, which unfortunately is impaired. When the person reaches an unexpected incline, the somatosensory system should be able to detect this; however, the soft carpeting and the patient's soft-soled shoes reduce the somatosensory information being relayed to the brain. In addition, because the inner ear balance system is impaired, the patient's "ears" do no tell him that he is tipping and a fall ultimately occurs. The patient did not realize he was tipping until it was too late because he could not sense the imbalance.

Another example illustrates the second reason for falling, **not being able to stop ourselves when tipping**. Imagine another person, age 85, walking down the isle of the same dark theater. This person's balance system is intact for all three systems, somatosensory, visual, and vestibular; however, this person's arms and legs are weak due to long-term inactivity, exacerbated by arthritis in the joints. When this person reaches the incline, he immediately notices it because of the excellent state of his vestibular and somatosensory balance systems. Sadly, however, even though this person is immediately aware that he is falling, he lacks the necessary strength and quickness in his legs to arrest the fall. This is an example of not being able to stop oneself once tipping.

Necessary Physical Attributes to Stop Falls

The second reason for falling stated above, that we cannot stop ourselves when tipping, indicates that we do not have the **strength, quickness, or coordination** to arrest the fall (Figure 3-1). If we could possess these attributes, many falls could be prevented.

Physiologic Requirements to Keep Us on Our Feet

In considering the physiologic requirements to keep us from falling, we first list the physical abilities we need to maintain our **upright stance** and then, stating these in the negative, list their negative counterparts. We need the following **four physiologic requirements** to keep us on our feet (Figure 3-2):

As seen in Figure 3-2, we need more than just good **balance** to maintain our upright stance. Without the necessary basic **strength**

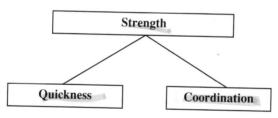

Figure 3–1. Desirable physical characteristics to stop falls.

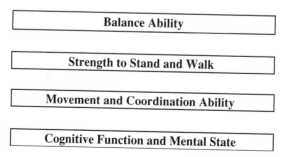

Figure 3–2. The four physiologic requirements for maintaining upright stance.

to stand and walk, we certainly will fall. Such is the case in persons with extreme frailty or weakness due to inactivity or disease. We also need basic **movement** and **coordination ability** lacking in some persons with neurologic or orthopedic disorders. Finally, without adequate mental ability, although we may be able to walk in a basic way, falls will be frequent if we lack the cognitive powers to perceive and avoid obstacles or dangerous situations. This is the case in advanced Alzheimer's disease, for example. Severe depression can have a similar effect.

Physiologic Dysfunctions That Lead to Falls

In the above section, we listed the physiologic requirements to keep us on our feet. Stated in the negative, the **four basic physiologic dysfunctions that lead to falls** are shown in Figure 3–3.

Regardless of the falls situation, no fall will occur if we can **sense that we are falling** as well as **stop the fall** before we hit the ground. For example, if we trip and begin to fall, we hopefully will recognize that we are falling but may not have the time necessary to prevent ourselves from hitting the ground. On the other hand, if we are unconscious and fall, we do not even sense that we were falling in the first place.

Center of Gravity and Base of Support

Another way of looking at falls theory is in terms of the body's "center of gravity." According to the laws of physics, we will fall when-

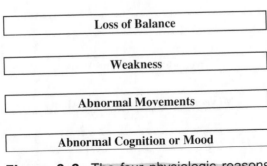

Loss of Balance

Weakness

Abnormal Movements

Abnormal Cognition or Mood

Figure 3–3. The four physiologic reasons for falls.

ever our "center of gravity" is not above our "base of support" (our legs and feet). However, even when such a situation occurs, a fall can sometimes be quickly averted by throwing out an arm or leg so that our center of gravity is now corrected and a possible fall avoided. This, of course, assumes that momentum is not too great, in which case the falling body may still continue its path to the ground. This "center of gravity" concept is an important one when we consider the various body types shown in Figure 3–4. As can be seen in these body types, somewhat more effort is constantly needed to keep these bodies from tipping over because these individuals are more likely to not have their centers of gravity over their base of support. If individuals with **off-centered body types** become weakened or otherwise incapacitated, their tendency to fall will be greater than persons with more symmetric body types.

In considering patients having body types such as those portrayed in Figure 3–4, it is often obvious why a person may be falling frequently. However, in many cases, just having a particular body type or physical characteristic is not the *main cause* of falls. Persons such as those shown in Figure 3–4 may have lived with their particular body type for years without falls, but when there is a new condition, such as a slightly impaired sensory balance system

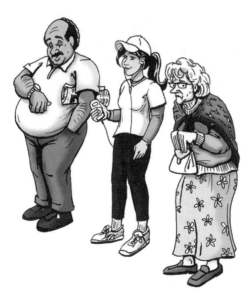

Figure 3–4. Body type can be a factor in maintaining center of gravity and avoiding falls.

or a weakened condition, this new situation results in frequent falls. **Despite the new abnormal balance condition, however, the patient may still be able to overcome the falls problem by strengthening, improving reaction times (quickness), or increasing coordination** if possible. This concept is particularly important when a medical condition such as decreased sense of balance cannot be completely resolved, as is sometimes the case.

Some examples may help to shed light on how various body types interact with other factors to cause falls.

Example 1

A patient says, "I lose my balance but because I am overweight and a little weak, I cannot help but fall."

This is an example of a person having a mild balance problem, along with other "extenuating circumstances," namely, being overweight so that the body is "harder to catch." Having weakened muscles to the point that there is not adequate strength to stop a fall is an additional factor leading to falls. But, although these circumstances make it harder to arrest falls, theoretically if the person had adequate strength and speed of leg reactions, stopping the fall would still be possible despite the minor balance disorder. In this case, the problem is that the person can sense that the body is falling, but the weight of the body is too great and the legs are too weak to stop the fall; therefore, the second problem mentioned above "**cannot stop ourselves when tipping**" is the **main cause** of the falls despite the balance problem. The extra weight and weaker muscles make it harder to stop a fall and could, therefore, be considered the principal causes of the falls instead of the balance problem, especially if these factors could be corrected.

Example 2

The patient is a 75-year-old male who is strong and has normal weight. However, the majority of his sense of balance is dysfunctional. This is due to the patient having partial dysfunction in each of the three balance systems, "legs," "eyes," and "inner ears." In this case, due to this patient's diabetes, he is partially blind and has some loss of feeling in his legs (peripheral neuropathy). He also was given an antibiotic recently that is ototoxic, resulting in some loss of inner ear balance (vestibular) on both sides. When standing on thick or soft carpeting, he often begins to tip forward, but because he cannot easily sense this tipping in any of the three balance systems until he has tipped too far, he does not realize this until it is too late. This case represents an example of the first possible reason for falling listed above, "**not realizing that we are tipping**." In order not to fall, we must realize that we are tipping before it is too late or, once tipping, we must have the extra strength and quickness necessary to stop the fall.

Determining the Main Reason for Falling

It is important in clinical practice to determine a patient's **main reason for falling** as opposed to simply calling the falls problem "multifactorial." Although several reasons often exist for falls, **determining the main cause is important in prioritizing the treatment or rehabilitation**. Calling a falls disorder "multifactorial" usually just means that the clinician cannot determine the true cause of the falls. In performing the falls examination at our clinic, we perform many tests to help determine the reasons a particular patient is falling. But, after all the data are gathered, we must look at the overall picture and ask "What is really causing this person to fall?" In asking this question, we must prioritize for rehabilitation the possible causes found during testing. For example, if a patient has only a slight decrease in balance ability, but is significantly weak in the knees and ankles and has the habit of rushing, these latter factors are identified as the most probable main cause. In the "falls assessment," we should not neglect to consider the more easily observable factors such as the patient's body type, other health problems, age, and personal habits. Quite often, the realization comes that if it were possible for patients to increase their **strength**, **quickness**, or **coordination**, there would be a much greater chance of arresting falls. For this reason, we often make recommendation for physical therapy, exercise, or other measures to accomplish these goals.

Fall Risk Factors

The causes of falls have often been divided into categories, such as "personal or environmental," "intrinsic or extrinsic." The term "intrinsic" refers to the fact that some falls are related mostly to the individual's personal status, be it medical, psychological, or behavioral, whereas other causes are related more to the environment, such as clutter on the floor ("extrinsic") (Stevens, 2005). We choose to classify falls as being **medical, behavioral,** or **environmental** (Table 3-1). Listing a separate category for "behavioral causes" emphasizes our belief, based on examination of many falling patients, that **behavioral factors play a large role in falls.** Many falls occur when persons are participating in activities or behaviors that are unwise from a falls safety standpoint. Safe behaviors are even more important when the balance ability is compromised as is the case in normal aging. Unfortunately, lifelong habits are difficult to break. For many people, standing on a step stool, carrying large loads while using the stairs, or rushing to answer the telephone or doorbell are unwise behaviors that are deeply ingrained. Because these actions are under the control of the individual (unless cognitively impaired), **falling is often as much a behavioral issue as a medical one.** Behavioral issues are covered in detail later.

We use the term "falls risk factors" to mean **any cause** of falls whether intrinsic or extrinsic; therefore, a cluttered home with many obstacles on the floor would be considered a "risk factor" just as having a medical condition causing falls would be a risk factor for that individual. We discuss each of the major risk factors in the following sections.

The common causes of falls are so varied that simply listing them is a challenging endeavor. Some causes are well recognized such as **imbalance, dizziness,** and **weakness,** whereas others are less common and less well understood as to their contribution to

Table 3–1. Causes of Falls

Medical		
Dizzy/Vertigo	Lightheaded/Faint	Balance Disorder
Behavioral		
Bad Habits	Personality	Psychological
Environmental		
Home	Work	Elsewhere

falls such as in **movement disorders** or **loss of consciousness** Table 3-2 lists many of the common as well as less common causes of falls that we encounter in the Falls Prevention Clinic at Henry Ford Hospital. Table 3-2 is only a partial list, but does demonstrate the wide variety of causes of falls and underscores the need for individual assessment.

Common Causes of Falls

An effective falls prevention program must include identification of the patient's medical as well as nonmedical causes of falling, prioritizing these causes, and then fitting the prevention strategies to the particular patient's situation. Identifying the causes of falls must include a thorough physical examination, included in the "falls examination," which requires a thorough understanding of the potential medical causes of falls.

Table 3–2. Causes of Falls

Common	Less Common
Dizziness or vertigo	Movement disorders
Imbalance	Poor coordination
Poor vision	Loss of consciousness
Dementia	
Weakness	Seizure
Blood pressure issues	Stroke
Cardiovascular factors (irregular heartbeat, etc.)	Heart attack
Neurological disorders	Abnormal gait, pain, or deformity of feet
Reduced feeling in the feet or legs (neuropathy)	Psychogenic
Environmental factors	Shoes
Behavioral factors	Depression

, Vertigo, or Loss of Balance

One of the most common causes of falls is dizziness, vertigo, or loss of balance. These terms are not synonymous. Patients having "balance problems" are those who either have a loss of a sense of balance (sensory disorder of the vestibular, somatosensory, or visual balance system) or have movement or coordination disorders. The latter disorders often are not related to disorders causing dizziness or vertigo, but are more often caused by stroke, neurologic, muscular, or orthopedic disorders. Patients who lose their balance but are not dizzy or vertiginous have a "balance problem" because they cannot move their bodies with sufficient accuracy or speed to maintain their stance or stop an impending fall. "Dizziness," on the other hand, is a vague term used loosely by both physicians and patients to mean anything from lightheadedness to true spinning "vertigo." Dizziness, in any of its forms, often leads to loss of balance sense and potential falls.

Poor Vision

Visual problems of various types including the use of new or improper prescriptive lenses are common causes of falls. Something as simple as wearing bifocals for the first time can cause falls because looking down through the "reading" section of the lenses causes the distance to the floor to seem distorted or "wrong." Problems as common as abnormal visual acuity or less common abnormal eye movements (oculomotor problem) can easily lead to falls. Older persons require much more light to achieve good vision. In such cases, adequate floor lighting is a crucial component of falls prevention. This is also the case when the vestibular balance system is impaired because, without the "inner ear" balance system, greater reliance is placed on the visual balance system. Neuro-ophthalmologists are physicians specializing in visual problems having a neurologic cause and serve as excellent consultants when a visual problem is not easily understood by the examiner. Neurologists are also familiar with unusual eye problems. For more common visual deficits, ophthalmologists or optometrists can provide assistance.

Dementia or Abnormal Consciousness

When we do not realize that we are in a state of imbalance or are tipping, it may be due to abnormal cognitive ability rather than simply a lack of balance sense. Persons with Alzheimer's disease, for example, have a much greater tendency to fall than others. An abnormal mental state may also be caused by medications or other chronic medical conditions.

A normal state of consciousness is also important to falls prevention. A certain amount of alertness is necessary to stand or walk safely. During unconsciousness, for example, we are usually not able to stand or walk, with sleepwalking being the exception (depending on the definition of "consciousness"). Mental alertness is required to avoid common obstacles while walking. Stated positively, falls and injury can often be avoided if there is adequate mental "presence of mind." Simply being distracted is a common cause of falls.

Weakness

If we are weak to the point that we lack the simple strength or body structure to maintain our stance, we will fall. Weakness, commonly found in the elderly or infirm, frequently leads to falls. For example, many persons of advanced age are considered to have **generalized body weakness**, or weakness in a part of the body necessary to maintain stance such as the lower extremities. Strength of the lower extremities should be tested clinically during the falls examination. Generalized body strength is sometimes estimated by determining the patient's hand grip strength. In our clinic, we rely mostly on determining the strength of the lower extremities.

Blood Pressure

Persons in the falls clinic frequently complain of being dizzy when they first stand up. This can be caused by a vestibular disorder or by a sudden drop in blood pressure on standing. **Postural hypotension**, defined as drop of 20 mm Hg in systolic blood pressure on standing after lying for 5 minutes (or a decrease to <90), causes falls because of the associated lightheadedness or near fainting (syncope).

Cardiovascular Factors

Cardiovascular conditions, such as rapid or slow heart rate (tachycardia or bradycardia), irregular heartbeat, as well as a variety of heart disorders can lead to feelings of dizziness, lightheadedness, or impending faint. Such conditions and their symptoms can occur in isolation; however, because they are more common in older individuals, these conditions often occur in combination with some of the other common medical conditions causing falls. "Cardiologists," trained as subspecialists in internal medicine, are best qualified to diagnose these conditions; however, internal medicine specialists are also trained to a significant extent in cardiology. Often, the patient can tell that his or her heart races at times, or has been told in the past by a physician that he or she has an irregular heartbeat. Although these conditions in isolation are not usually the primary cause of falls, because they are so common, these are considered common possible "contributors" to falls. Fortunately, cardiovascular disorders are frequently controlled by medications but patients are sometimes taking two or three medications that affect their blood pressure or cardiovascular status which therefore should be considered.

Neurologic Disorders

Neurologic disorders that can affect balance commonly lead to falls. Such disorders include Parkinsonism, various forms of ataxia (gait disorder), strokes, and tumors causing damage to the balance areas of the nervous system such as the cerebellum as well as other degenerative diseases. Neurologic disorders can be of sudden onset, such as in stroke, or have a very gradual onset such as in Parkinson's disease. Disorders that are of gradual onset are difficult to diagnose both in terms of whether or not a disorder even exists or whether the symptoms are just a sign of "normal" aging. For example, a shuffling or slow gait with gradually decreasing balance can be a sign of Parkinson's disease or just simple aging. Only when such disorders are having a greater effect are they easily recognized. During the period of mild symptoms, however, falls may be common. The question of whether or not physical therapy or exercise may benefit such individuals is often a difficult one. It is usually best to err on the side of trying exercise; however, any exercise with such patients must be safe, which means there must be something stable to hold onto such as an exercise bar, walker, or stable shopping cart.

Reduced Feeling in the Feet or Legs (Neuropathy)

Reduced feeling in the feet or legs, often due to "peripheral neuropathy," is a common major contributor to falls. The lack of sensation in the feet, for example, causes a person to not correctly sense the floor. Often, the individual with neuropathy will describe the sensation of walking on marshmallows or pillows. Lacking adequate feeling in the feet makes it difficult to sense whether the floor is slanted, slippery, or stable. This disorder also may affect the somatosensory or proprioceptive systems, which let us know "by feel" what our legs or other limbs are doing. Patients with neuropathy of the lower extremities require the use of vision to a greater extent to discern correctly the location of the feet in relation to the floor.

As with the vertiginous or visually deficient patients, adequate floor lighting is a critical falls prevention measure.

Environmental Factors

Environmental factors leading to falls have been termed "extrinsic," in that they occur due to factors outside the individual. All of us are familiar with obstacles on the floor causing trips and falls; however this issue is more important for an individual who is already prone to falling. Persons with decreased vision, inability to quickly react, or those more susceptible to injury such as the aged, are at even greater danger from environmental factors. Not only are obstacles a problem but a host of environmental issues exist that should be considered. Discussing and considering these environmental factors becomes one of the major activities during falls prevention efforts. Lists of danger factors in the home or other dangerous situations are often presented to potential fallers. Included in such lists are recommendations for the installation of grab bars, hand rails, bedside commodes, the removal of throw rugs, as well as other important measures aimed at preventing falls. Home inspections are also sometimes appropriately recommended, which may result in internal modifications to the living environment. In extreme cases, where there are dangerous situations and where there is little outside help available or family support, recommendation is made for the patient to move. It is our belief, however, that keeping the individual in his or her own familiar environment is usually more appropriate. More about the environmental aspects of falls prevention is presented in Chapter 6.

Behavioral Factors

In our experience, behavioral factors play a major part in the occurrence of falls. We frequently hear from our off-balance patients that they use step stools, rush to answer the door or phone, walk alone outside at night, as well as engage in a number of other risky behaviors. Old habits are hard to break, but sometimes patients will also do something that they know is unwise for emotional reasons, such as hoping to prove to themselves or others that they still have the skills they need to live independently. Chapter 6. has information on the behavioral aspects of falls, including suggested methods for modifying risky behaviors. Related to behavioral factors are possible **psychogenic causes**, although these are rare (see section on psychogenic causes below).

Less Common Causes of Falls

Some less common causes of falling are summarized in Table 3–2.

Movement and Mobility Disorders

A mobility problem consists of the inability to move the body appropriately. Even though our sense of balance and ability to maintain stance may be normal, if we lack the ability to move our body properly and perform the minor adjustments needed to maintain our balance, we will fall more easily. Movement disorders, stiffness in the legs, orthopedic problems, abnormal body weight, as well as a host of other factors affect mobility and coordination.

The term **movement disorder** refers to a motor impairment resulting in an inability to move the body properly. For our purposes, movement disorder does not refer to an impairment in the sensory "balance system." Movement disorders can cause falls when the ability to walk with a normal gait is impaired. Frequent tripping, stumbling, or shuffling of the feet understandably can cause falls. A well-trained eye is necessary to distinguish between an abnormal gait caused by a movement disorder and one caused by a balance system disorder. Movement disorders usually manifest themselves not just while walking but also while seated and attempting to move the limbs, such as when asked to perform basic cerebellar tests of coordination.

Orthopedic problems such as deformity or pain can also cause inaccurate or inefficient movements leading to falls. Adequate **range of motion**, which is the ability of an extremity to move easily the full distance necessary to perform the needed action, is also needed to prevent falls. The full range of motion seen in younger individuals may not be needed to prevent falls, but significantly **limited range of motion**, such as that caused by knee, hip, or ankle disorders is certainly detrimental to safe ambulation. Physical therapists are experienced in assessing range of motion and making recommendations for possible improvement.

Poor Coordination

Occasionally, patients will present to the Falls Prevention Clinic who have been known to have poorer than average coordination throughout their lives. Although this may be true, care should be taken to ensure that such patients do not have a long-standing balance disturbance such as benign positional vertigo that is being mistaken for an innate lifelong balance problem. All patients arriving with the history of "lifelong lack of coordination" should receive at least a **vestibular and balance screening**. When the case is truly one of lifelong subaverage coordination, it may become increasingly worse due to aging and lead to falls.

Loss of Consciousness

Complete loss of consciousness, although relatively rare, can be due to a wide variety of medical conditions, including serious conditions such as stroke, seizure, or other catastrophic medical events. Less serious conditions, such as severe postural hypotension or vasovagal reaction, also can cause loss of consciousness. Near loss of consciousness is also a risk factor for falls. Patients often will often claim to have lost consciousness when they are ultimately found to have a vestibular disorder or other condition unlikely to cause loss of consciousness. Vertigo can be a very upsetting feeling when it first occurs, and some patients will report this as "passing out" especially if a fall occurs. The complaint of passing out should not discourage the clinician from looking into the possibility of inner ear-induced vertigo as the correct etiology of the fall.

Seizure, Stroke, or Heart Attack-Induced Collapse

Catastrophic medical conditions such as seizure, stroke, or heart attack may lead to a fall due to the collapse of the patient. Such episodes are difficult to predict and prevent. Vigilance on the part of patient caretakers, family, and close associates also is important, and there should be a plan in place should such an event occur. The environment of such a potential victim should be free of objects that may be fallen upon causing injury which can be more severe than the medical event itself.

Abnormal Gait, Pain, or Deformity of Feet or Legs

Abnormal gait is associated with falls in the aging population (Montero-Odasso et al., 2005). Gait problems can be caused by a variety of musculoskeletal, neurologic and even psychological problems. The purpose of gait assessment for the falls clinic evaluation is concerned not only with diagnosis but, more importantly, also from the standpoint of assessing what effect the abnormal gait may have on falls risk. A major issue is determining whether the person would be safe while walking without an assistive device. It is at this point in the examination that the need for a walker or cane is often determined. An approach that is often effective in recommending a walker is that this device will aid the person in remaining independent longer. The topic of assistive devices is covered in Chapter 6.

Common gait abnormalities seen in falls patients are **wide-based gait** often seen in vestibular disorders (the patient walks with legs farther apart to compensate for the lack of a finely tuned vestibular balance system); **halting gait**, in which the patient's speed of walking is not smooth and continuous; **deviating gait**, in which the patient staggers or drifts to the left or right; and **rapid gait**. A rapid gait can result from the patient being able to balance better when walking quickly than when walking more slowly similar to the way in which it is more difficult to ride a bicycle at an extremely slow speed. Although an attempt is often made to slow down gait that is too rapid, this approach may backfire because the person may need to walk slightly faster to keep balance. In many cases, however, a person walks quickly simply because he or she has a personality to do things quickly. Such a person will claim to have always been a "rusher" throughout his or her life. The examiner can simply ask whether this is the case or whether the person walks quickly in order to keep better balance.

Gait can be assessed using the descriptors of Tinetti (1994) whose concepts are briefly summarized in Chapter 2. More details on how to utilize the Tinetti criteria for gait assessment are covered in Chapter 5, Falls Examination.

Helping a patient to alter his or her walking pattern may be a means of reducing falls risk if the abnormal gait is not too severe. Altering the gait is often more a behavioral modification issue (see Chapter 6). In this regard, we have developed "SafeWalk" techniques in which the patient is taught new, safer walking techniques that are designed to avoid falls. These include developing the habits of avoiding rapid head turns while walking, turning corners too quickly, or carrying things in both hands. Chapter 6 discusses these techniques.

Musculoskeletal problems cause or contribute to falls. For example, foot pain is a common cause of reduction in exercise and development of abnormal gait. Foot disorders can cause falls directly due to deformity or dysfunction or indirectly by reducing the amount of exercise a person receives because of foot pain or other abnormality. Pain in the feet can cause a person to have an abnormal gait that causes a person to walk in such a way as to avoid pain. Efforts should focus on the underlying causes of the pain which can be due to a wide variety of foot and leg issues. Podiatrists are good resources in cases of foot pain, which can result from as simple a cause as long or ingrown toenails or other more serious disorder. Orthopedic surgeons are highly qualified to assess and treat major deformities of the legs.

Arthritis of the lower extremities as well as disorders of the neck or back are potential causes of abnormal gait. Arthritis in the knees is common in older individuals and may sometimes cause a deformity in which the foot is "out toe'd" (i.e., pointed constantly outward when walking). This problem can cause falls due to the foot catching on obstacles while walking. An ongoing study at Henry Ford hospital is exploring the incidence of knee abnormality contributing to falls.

Shoes

Sometimes an aging, falling individual will resort to thick-soled athletic shoes for falls prevention. A well-meaning relative may also provide and encourage the use of such shoes because of the benefits of the improved traction. Two problems may occur with such a recommendation. Shoes with thicker soles than the patient is used to catch more easily on the floor because the patient is standing slightly higher, which makes the floor seem lower from the patient's visual perspective. Athletic shoes often also have soles made of softer rubber, which, although less likely to slip, may stick and catch more easily on the floor. Patients wearing athletic shoes often report catching their toe on the carpet or floor more easily. Normally, switching the type of shoes patients are used to is not a wise idea unless there are glaring problems, such as the use of extremely high heels or shoes completely lacking support. In the case of sandals, house shoes, or slippers without backs, such loose footwear frequently causes falls. On the other hand, slightly high heels may actually prevent falls if they are not loose and the patient is used to them. Some patients comment that their balance seems better in such shoes, which is probably due to the fact that the heel causes a forward slant to the patient's posture. As many older patients have a tendency to fall backward, a moderately small heel may help prevent falls.

Depression

It is not known the extent to which depression is a factor in falls; however, depression is known to sometimes cause a decrease in the level of cognitive function, which itself is known to cause falls. The apparent abnormal cognitive function of some individuals is sometimes really depression disguised as abnormal cognition. Neuropsychologists are well suited to evaluate such cases in detail. Simple screening measures for both cognition and depression should always be part of falls examinations.

Psychogenic Causes

Although rare, severe psychogenic disorders may cause a person to fall, due to erratic behavior, lack of judgment, or the ill effects on cognition that severe depression can cause.

Other Medical Conditions

Most falls are related to the **nervous, musculoskeletal**, or **cardio-vascular** systems; however, under the "wrong" circumstances, it is possible for nearly any body system or subsystem to cause or contribute to falls. For example, falls can be caused by a deficit in the respiratory system such as in hypoxia with resultant disorientation, lightheadedness, or syncope.

Aging Changes in Ability to React Quickly

As a younger person responds to a slip, sudden compensatory movements occur in the hips and ankles to prevent the fall. As we get older, however, more emphasis is placed on taking a rapid step ahead, or moving an arm or leg to prevent the fall. Unfortunately the ability to effectively use these strategies decreases with age. There is also slowed reaction time, decreased alertness, and lower muscle strength. Lesser (2006) notes that older individuals also have increased sway in their gait, particularly after a hip fracture that could contribute to falls.

Studies by Other Authors on Causes of Falls

Other authors have also reported common "causes of falls." Each of these articles lists some factors in common, but some factors are listed only in a single study. Rubenstein and Josephson (2002) have summarized the causes of falls as reported in the geriatric literature.

In order of importance, the top causes included **accident and environment-related** (31%), **gait and balance disorders or weakness** (17%), **other** (15%), **dizziness and vertigo** (13%), **drop attack** (9%), **confusion** (5%), **unknown** (5%), **postural hypotension** (3%), **visual** (2%), and **syncope** (0.3%). These percentages are approximate because the "other" and "unknown" categories also contain some medical or environmental causes. From these figures, we can extrapolate that **all medically related issues combined constitute the greatest category of falls causes (total 49%)**, with environmental causes also contributing significantly (31%). Further consideration of these data suggests that audiologists are well suited to falls prevention as a significant percentage of falls (30%) are attributed to dizziness and balance-related causes, which many audiologists assess. Lesser (2006) cites a recent study stating that of 428 elderly patients who fell without known cause, 80% had symptoms of vestibular impairment in the past year that could have contributed to their falls.

Notwithstanding the causes listed above, other studies differ in reported falls risk factors. Table 3–3 lists risk factors noted by various authors. Factors listed in bold represent risk factors that were not listed in Table 3–2 nor discussed above.

Myriad Risk Factors

It is apparent from these articles that there are a multiplicity of fall risk factors. This underscores the need for individual assessment. Although most reported risk factors are understandable, some are surprising. For example, it is not obvious why the use of four or more medications correlates to falling; however, some possible reasons are **drug interactions** plus the likelihood that with four medications, some are likely to affect blood pressure or have a sedating side effect. A high percentage of medications list "dizziness" as a possible side effect. Also, the reduced physical condition that is likely to be present in someone using four or more medications may be a predisposing factor.

Reduced **arm muscle strength**, or "**grip strength**," is another surprising risk factor; however, this probably relates to falling because grip strength is an indirect measure of general body strength, which is known to be associated with falling.

Table 3–3. Falls Risk Factors Noted by Various Authors*

Rubenstein and Josephson (2002)	Jacobson (2002)
accident and environment-related (31%)	decreased cognitive function
	increased reaction time
gait and balance disorders or weakness (17%)	depression (and associated medications)
other (15%)	postural hypotension
dizziness and vertigo (13%)	impaired proprioception
drop attack (9%)	**impaired postural stability**
confusion (5%)	impairments having effect on postural control such as hemiparesis and paraplegia
unknown (5%)	
postural hypotension (3%)	Parkinson's disease
visual (2%)	impaired balance function
syncope (0.3%)	impaired visual function
	four or more medications
Stevens (2005)	difficulty transferring
old age	environmental hazards
history of falls	impaired gait
being female	impaired arm muscle strength or range of motion
lower body weakness	
problems with gait and balance	**Tinetti et al. (1994)**
taking four or more medications of any type	**prescription of four or more medications**
any psychoactive medication	**inability to transfer safely from tub or toilet**
vision impairment	environmental hazards for falls or tripping
certain chronic diseases such as Parkinson's	
history of stroke	impairment of gait
arthritis	**impairment in arm muscle strength or range of motion**

continues

59

Table 3–3. *continued*

Tinetti, Doucette, Claus, and Marotolli (1995) (risk factors independently associated with **serious injury** after falls): **low body mass** **female gender** balance and gait impairment **presence of at least two chronic conditions** cognitive impairment	Blake et al. (1988) **use of hypnotics or antidepressants** **handgrip strength in the dominant hand** **symptoms of arthritis** giddiness foot difficulties

*Boldface factors are not listed in Table 3-2 and were not discussed previously in this chapter.

Why the Difference Between Studies?

The difference in reported risk factors may be due, in part, to difficulties in determining the actual cause of the falls in the patients that were studied. For example, in some studies, it is the physician who determines the cause of the fall after speaking with and assessing the patient. Other studies ask for the patient's opinion. In a study by Blake, Morgan, Bendall, et al. (1988), 1042 individuals aged 65 years and older, were interviewed, 35% of whom had experienced falls in the preceding year. When asked to give the reason for their falls, 53% simply reported "tripping" and 19% could not give a reason. From this we learn that, because there must be some cause of the frequent "tripping," many people cannot ascertain the underlying cause of their own falls.

Tinetti, Inouye, Gill, and Doucette (1995) reported several more risk factors in terms of "**relative risk**," which quantified the risk associated with each factor. These included performance ability on various practical tests. Among the factors found to put a patient most at risk included **abnormal score on an informal balance test, slow in ability to stand from sitting consecutively three times** (>10 seconds), **slowed gait when attempting to walk quickly, slowed ability to tap the foot ten times**

(>6.6 seconds), **abnormal Mini-Mental Status Score** (<20), **arm strength impairment, insulin use, and slowed usual gait speed**. Other interesting factors putting a patient at greater than normal risk of falling were abnormally slow signature speed, self-rated poor health, incontinence, and age 80 or older. More about tests for predicting falls in a given individual are given in Chapters 5 and 7.

As discussed above, some of the risk factors were significant in one study but not mentioned in another. However, the above results are often based on averages; therefore, it should not be assumed that the factors not found to be significant in one study are not significant in certain individuals. To the contrary, it is well known that some factors having a low relative risk certainly do cause falls in some individuals, particularly if the amount of the factor is high enough. For example, **antihypertensives**, at too high dose or in wrong combinations in some individuals are a cause of postural hypotension-induced syncope. High **body mass in combination with low leg strength** is certainly also a risk factor. **Previous stroke** can cause permanent damage that leads to future falls, and **arthritis**, if significant, can reduce flexibility of ankles, knees, and hips or cause pain while ambulating, thus causing falls.

The "Guidelines of the Prevention of Falls in Older Persons," a joint document by the American Geriatrics Society, British Geriatrics Society, and American Academy of Orthopedic Surgeons Panel on Falls Prevention (2001), specifically mentions **arthritis** and the **use of an assistive device** (cane or walker) as significant risk factors in addition to some of those already mentioned. Although canes and walkers certainly prevent falls in many individuals, in others, they do not prevent falls and may even be the cause of falls. In some individuals, the legs tend to get tangled in a cane or walker, thus causing falls. This underscores the need for an individual assessment that includes observing the patient using the device when recommending canes or walking aids.

The use of **exercise**, as discussed in more detail in Chapter 6 on falls prevention, also is controversial at the present time because there are patients for whom more exercise actually causes a greater number of falls. This is because persons who begin an exercise program move around more and, in doing so, put themselves at risk. Generally speaking, if exercise is safe, which means the patient has something to hold onto, the greater strength and flexibility obtained by the participant is beneficial in reducing falls and their associated injuries.

Other Factors

There are other risk factors not stressed in the previous literature that certainly lead to falls such as **deformity of the lower extremities**, **pain when walking** causing abnormal gait, as well as various less common **neurologic or motor disorders**. A wide **variety of medications** increase falls risk with a high percentage of medications listing vertigo, dizziness, imbalance, or falling as possible adverse reactions. Hypnotics, pain, or sedating medications particularly add falls risk as do some of the anti-seizure medications, which are significantly disruptive of normal balance. **Ototoxic medications** cause either hearing or balance problems or both. These include many aminoglycosides, chemotherapeutic drugs, and others including Quinine, which has in recent years become popular again for leg cramps. The bilaterally reduced vestibular response, that such ototoxic drugs can cause, lessens or obliterates the sensitivity of the vestibular balance system. Finally, in keeping with the behavior-based theme of this book, having certain **behavioral patterns**, such as being a "rusher" or "risk taker," also predisposes a person to falls.

Risk of Serious Injury

Tinetti, Doucette, Claus, and Marotelli (1995) reported risk factors associated with serious injury after falls. These risk factors were **low body mass**, being **female**, **balance and gait impairment**, **presence of at least two chronic conditions**, and **cognitive impairment**. These factors were "independently" associated with injury risk, that is, any one of them poses a risk.

Tests for Determining Individual Risk

Perhaps the most compelling question facing those working with the elderly is, "How can I recognize the person who is likely to fall." This is where the concept of simple performance tests comes in.

In some settings at least, the practical goal is to determine who is at high risk so that these individuals may be prioritized for intervention. Luckily, there are such tests available. These are covered in Chapter 7, which covers patients in hospitals and nursing homes. Such tests are often based on a patient's performance while walking, turning, or performing other tasks. It is logical that having the person walk, turn, or perform functions that tax the patient's abilities will help determine the extent of risk of falling. Again, simply identifying risk factors is not practical, because there are so many factors that few older individuals will not have at least some "risk factors" for falls. In fact, multiple risk factors in a given aging individual are the norm not the exception. This situation makes the evaluation of the cause of falling in a given individual complex; however, as outlined in Chapter 5 describing the Falls Clinic (Chapter 5), determining the main cause of falls is usually achievable.

Common Fall Types

Imagine a young healthy individual walking down a sidewalk. Balance is maintained by the three balance systems, visual ("eyes" and related structures), somatosensory ("leg balance system" mainly in the lower extremities), and vestibular ("inner ear" and related structures (see Chapter 2). Fortunately, we can learn to keep our balance even if we lose one of these systems completely. For example, some deaf individuals also lose their inner ear balance system completely at the time their hearing is lost. Over time (usually a few months), the visual and somatosensory balance systems compensate to a great extent in these individuals, although some of the "fine tuning" of balance may be permanently lost. For example, individuals without vestibular balance may notice reduced balance ability in dimly lit areas where the visual system cannot be utilized. Of course, in addition to the balance systems, we also need good muscle coordination and movement ability to keep our balance while walking.

From the previous discussion, it is easy to see that there are many possible causes of imbalance and falls. This book has focused on the many medical and extrinsic causes of falls in other chapters. It is useful to think of falls in terms of various "**fall types**" to properly rehabilitate the falling patient. Some of the most common "fall types" are summarized below. Understanding the general etiologies of these fall types is helpful when differentiating the cause, and therefore the proper rehabilitation strategy, for these falls. The final example consists of a case having a combination of the "fall types." However, even in the combination cases, it is nevertheless important to determine the "main cause" of falling so that rehabilitation can be prioritized toward the main cause.

Falls Type 1: "I don't realize I am falling"

Persons having a loss of sensory input from one of the balance systems (see Chapter 2) may not realize that they are falling until it is too late to arrest the fall. A good question to differentiate this problem is, "When you fall, do you realize you are tipping?" These patients may say, "I don't know I am falling until I end up on the ground (or nearly on the ground)." Although such a claim may be due to a loss of sensory balance information such as in a vestibular, visual, or somatosensory balance disorder, this complaint may occasionally be present in persons with syncope (fainting) or loss of consciousness due to seizure or stroke.

Falls Type 2: "I know that I am falling but I can't help it"

Persons who have a loss of mobility (ability to move or coordinate the limbs) or are generally weaker than needed for their body size often realize they are tipping but are nearly helpless to do anything about it. Such persons may lack either the quickness, strength, or coordination to stop a fall, or they may be too weak generally. In differentiating between the balance problem of the first example and this example, it is often helpful to ask the patient, "Do you think that it is your legs or your balance that is the problem." Some patients can ascertain this difference; others cannot. If persons are weak or otherwise lack the ability to stop a fall, they often are aware of this. Therefore, asking the patient's opinion is often an important aspect of ascertaining the true main cause of falls.

Falls Type 3: "I don't know why I fall"

Some persons cannot seem to give any information relating to their falls. When pressed, they give the impression of someone who was not aware of the fall until hitting the ground. If asked if they were unconscious, they may not know. In some cases, this inability to give any information is due to a reduced cognitive ability. "I just find myself on the floor" is a common comment by such individuals. The examiner must be careful not to mistake such comments for those of a person with normal cognition who is simply expressing the surprising unexpected nature of their falls. Syncope, seizure, or cardiogenic disorders occasionally are causes of not knowing why a fall occurred; however, in our experience, such expressions are frequently made by persons having vestibular or other common balance problems, particularly in those of advanced age.

Falls Type 4: "Combination of causes"

In this example the combination is one of a loss of sense of body position, plus a movement disorder.

This patient while walking does not feel that he is tipping, and then, when he does, is not capable of quickly moving his body into a position that will prevent the fall. His combination of the lack of the balance sense, as seen in vestibular disorder, plus a generalized body weakness, which is often seen in the elderly, spells disaster in the form of dangerous falls.

According to many patients we have examined, this is one of the most common types of falls, occurring mainly while the patient is simply walking (not climbing stairs, tripping, or bending). While standing or walking, our musculoskeletal system is constantly making small adjustments to keep our body erect based on information obtained from our visual (eyes), somatosensory (legs and related structures), and vestibular (inner ear and related structures) balance systems. More simply stated, if we "feel" ourselves tipping, we make the automatic adjustments necessary to keep our balance. The problem occurs when we tip farther than usual. This may be termed the "**critical fall angle**," which differs among individuals based on many factors such as body height, weight, shape, and strength issues. When our body tips off-center beyond this certain critical angle, a strong and rapid correction is necessary to keep our balance, such as taking a strong, quick step forward to catch ourselves. When such a reaction does not happen quickly enough or with enough force, our body will continue to tip and we find ourselves on the floor. In older individuals, additional problems may occur which slow the sensory messages as well as the needed muscle responses. There is often poor vision, weaker muscle sensations, or reduced ear balance input to the extent that the message that we are tipping is received too slowly or not at all. "All I know is that I was suddenly on the floor," is a typical description of falls by an older person. In addition, older individuals often have weaker muscles and slower reaction times. The ability to throw the foot out is slower and the muscular response is weaker once the foot gets there.

During walking, and especially while turning, the problem becomes even more exaggerated as the speed at which we are moving adds momentum and force to our moving body, which must be overcome by the restoring forces just mentioned. Just as a speeding car can turn too quickly and roll over, a body moving quickly can also turn so quickly as not to be able to overcome the forces causing it to tip.

Inability to catch ourselves when tipping off center, due either to our being less aware of tipping, having slower reaction times, or having inadequate strength to stop the fall, represents a large percentage of falls presenting to our clinic.

Strong, Quick, and Coordinated

Going back to the principles put forth in the beginning of the chapter, more than just good balance is required to prevent falls. Being **strong** enough to prevent a fall, **quick** enough to respond to tipping before it is too late, and **coordinated** enough to properly counteract the falling body are attributes of successful nonfallers. On the other hand, being **weak**, **slow**, and **uncoordinated** are common attributes of frequent fallers. Improving one or more of these attributes is often an effective way to prevent falls. Working to improve these three physical "Falls-Proof" attributes is worthy of our significant efforts in preventing falls. Reaction times may be improved through practice by using activities such as sports or indoor games that require quick movements. Improving strength and flexibility can be accomplished even in the elderly by utilizing weight-bearing exercise. Again, safe exercise requires the ability to hold onto something while exercising such as using a shopping cart.

Admittedly, other attributes can affect the tendency to fall. For example, if a person is extremely overweight, then muscles even of "normal strength" may still not be adequate to maintain balance when tipping. Another attribute, flexibility, is also necessary in addition to having adequate strength; therefore, stretching activities should not be forgotten when trying to improve strength.

Having good balance **sensitivity** is also important to falls prevention. Sensory balance sensitivity can be improved by increasing visual sensitivity through increased lighting, placing colored tape at the edges of steps, or using corrective vision lenses. Vestibular rehabilitation exercises are important in many cases for improving vestibular sensitivity and function. This rehabilitation is offered by many audiologists or physical therapists.

Somatosensory problems, which affect the ability to determine where the legs are and what they are doing, is often difficult to rehabilitate but sometimes this problem can be helped somewhat through physical therapy. Sometimes a simple loose elastic bandage at the knees will help with somatosensory sensation.

Summary

This chapter presented a "theory of falling" and gave examples of each of the conditions leading to falls as well as "risk factors." We have observed too great a tendency among clinicians to simply attribute a patient's falls problem to "multifactorial" causes without prioritizing the causes or attempting to identify the "main causes" of falls in an individual. It is hoped that an understanding of the factors presented in this chapter will allow the clinician to effectively evaluate each individual's situation in light of what can be done to improve the situation. It is the philosophy of this text that most falls can be prevented if motivation exists and the patient is capable of adapting. By understanding the principles presented in this chapter, clinicians and patients may more effectively achieve this goal.

References

American Geriatrics Society, British Geriatrics Society, B and American Academy of Orthopaedic Surgeons Panel on Falls Prevention. (2001). Guidelines for the prevention of falls in older persons. *Journal of the American Geriatric Society, 49,* 664.

Blake A. J., Morgan, K., Bendall, M. J., Dallosso H, Ebrahim, S. B., Arie, T. H., et al. (1988). Falls by elderly people at home: Prevalence and associated factors. *Age and Ageing, 17*, 365-372.

Jacobson, G. P. (2002). Development of a clinic for the assessment of risk of falls in elderly patients. *Seminars in Hearing 23*(2), 161-178.

Lesser, T. H. J. (2006). Elderly fallers and the ENT surgeon. *ENT News, 15*(1), 59-60.

Montero-Odasso, M., Schapira, M., Duque, G., Soriano, E. R., Kaplan, R., & Camera, L. A. (2005). Gait disorders are associated with non-cardiovascular falls in elderly people: A preliminary study. *BMC Geriatrics, 1*(5), 15.

Rubenstein, L. Z., & Josephson, K. R. (2002). The epidemiology of fall and syncope. *Clinical Geriatric Medicine, 18*, 146.

Stevens, J. A. (2005). Falls among older adults: Risk factors and prevention strategies. *Journal of Safety Research, 26*(4), 409-411.

Tinetti, M. E., Baker, D. I., McAvay, G., Claus, E. B., Garrett, P., Gottschalk, M., et al. (1994). A multifactorial intervention to reduce the risk of falling among elderly people living in the community. *New England Journal of Medicine, 331*, 821-827.

Tinetti, M. E., Doucette, J., Claus, E., & Marottoli, R. (1995). Risk factors for serious injury during falls by older persons in the community. *Journal of the American Geriatric Society, 43*(11), 1214-1221.

Tinetti, M. E., Inouye, S. K., Gill, T. M., & Doucette, J. T. (1995). Shared risk factors for falls, incontinence and functional independence. *Journal of the American Medical Association, 273*(17), 1348-1353.

CHAPTER 4

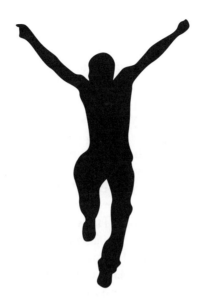

Dizziness as a Symptom

The complaint of "dizziness" is so common that it deserves a chapter of its own. Although the topic is also discussed elsewhere in the book, this chapter is meant to provide an introduction for both the professional who is either less involved or new to the topic as well as the layman who may desire a general overview. There are at least two reasons for discussing dizziness separately. First, the term dizziness is so commonly misused and misunderstood. Second, because there is such a great diversity among the causes of "dizziness," each should be discussed in detail. The main purpose of this short chapter is to compare the terms "dizziness," "vertigo," and "lightheaded" with other terms that are sometimes substituted or confused with them.

What Does the Term Dizziness Mean?

Unfortunately, the term "dizzy" means different things to different people, even within the medical field. Among the general population, especially in a bygone era, the term "dizzy" was also used to connote a mentally confused state, for example, the term "you're dizzy" meant "you're crazy." It is fair to say, however, that in today's world the term "dizzy" does not usually connote an abnormal mental state or personality trait, but unfortunately is used to signify a wide variety of medical symptoms including true vertigo, light-headedness, disorientation, mental confusion, impending faint, weakness, impaired vision, heart palpitations, as well as others. The term "dizzy" is so commonly used, that one emergency room's softball team known to the author, called themselves the "WADAOs," meaning "weak and dizzy all over" to signify the phrase heard quite often from their patients. Fortunately, most medical professionals are more specific in their designation of symptoms and use the term "dizziness" infrequently. In making these distinctions, medical professionals usually differentiate vertigo as a patient's complaint of a "spinning sensation" referring to either the patient or his or her surroundings. Although the question "does the room spin?" is usually a good one for determining this, in many cases, the patient finds it difficult to answer with certainty. Especially when symptoms are mild or vague, patients express frustration at not being able to describe the feeling they are experiencing. In such cases, it is best not to prompt the patient with potential descriptors; but rather to ask open ended questions like "how do you feel?"

In the following sections, each of the descriptors often used by patients or health care providers when describing their symptoms are discussed along with some of the common causes for each.

Vertigo

Vertigo, which is defined as a "hallucination of movement," is most frequently described as a "spinning sensation." Vertigo is sometimes referred to as "true vertigo," signifying that the examiner has determined the symptom to be one of motion as opposed to a feeling of lightheadedness, disorientation, or other sensation in which there is no component of motion. The problem with requiring that the component of motion be included is that, particulary in its milder forms when the "inner ear" is the cause, there is often not a true feeling of motion. Rather, patients often will say, "I don't feel like I am actually moving or things around me are moving, but I feel as though I have just come off a ride at an amusement park, as though I had been moving." Sometimes patients may say that, in the beginning, they felt as if they were moving or spinning, but they no longer feel the symptoms so severely. Often the comment is, "I am just a little off, especially when I move my head quickly or in certain ways." Such descriptions should be included in the designation "vertigo," or at least under the heading of those disorders that cause vertigo, especially if there was once a true feeling of spinning. Holding to the requirement of a feeling of movement would, in the author's opinion, exclude the largest percentage of patients with true vestibular disorders (inner ear), especially because the two most common vestibular disorders are benign paroxysmal positional vertigo (BPPV) and vestibular neuritis. These two disorders can both present with mild symptoms in the office, with more frank vertigo showing itself only when subjecting the patient to a provoking maneuver such as the Dix-Hallpike or "head shake" tests.

Causes of Vertigo

The most common causes of true vertigo are vestibular, with more serious central nervous system causes ("central") being less frequent. The most common vestibular disorders causing either frank vertigo or the "slightly off" feeling described above include benign paroxysmal positional vertigo (BPPV), vestibular neuritis (sometimes called vestibular "neuronitis"), perilymph fistula, superior semicircular canal dehiscence, viral labrynthitis, sudden sensorineural hearing loss, Ménière's disease, and ototoxicity due to medications. More information on some of these topics is given elsewhere in this book (Chapters 2 and 5).

Lightheadedness

Lightheadedness or a feeling of impending faint, is sometimes difficult for the patient to differentiate from the milder forms of vertigo mentioned above. This symptom is due to a reduced function in awareness centers of the brain.

Causes of Lightheadedness

Lightheadedness can be caused by a wide variety of disorders, including reduction in blood flow, toxicity due to disease or external substances, reduced oxygenation to the brain, trauma, and intracranial lesions. Most common causes are blood pressure issues and cardiogenic causes such as irregular heart rate.

Off Balance

The symptom of "off balance" is a vague term usually used by patients to describe abnormal walking ability. "I stagger like a drunk," "I am always bumping into walls," or "people tell me I veer to the side" are frequent comments. Patients also may substitute the term "off balance" when they are actually feeling vertigo. Most professionals reserve the term "abnormal balance" to signify a patient's inability to maintain steadiness when walking or standing that is observable to the examiner. Although patients with vestibular vertigo may also be "off balance," patients with exclusive "balance disorders" that are neurologically based generally do not feel symptoms when only sitting or lying down.

Balance disorders are most commonly due to either a loss of sensory input or abnormal processing of the input by one of the three balance systems (visual, somatosensory, or vestibular; see Chapter 2), but may also be due to abnormal ability to respond to that input. For example, a patient with a **movement disorder** may realize he is falling, but is not able to do anything about it, the response of the legs being either too slow or too inaccurate to stop the fall.

Causes of "Off Balance"

Exclusive "balance" disorders (not caused by vertigo) may denote serious neurologic problem (Parkinson's disease, poststroke, etc.); however, a variety of "lesser" conditions can also result in imbalance. Other common disorders causing imbalance include lower back problems, orthopedic disorders of the lower extremities, lack of sensation in the legs or feet (neuropathy), arthritis, pain when walking, foot disorders, and medications. In addition, generalized body weakness is a common problem in the elderly that can be due to disease, deconditioning, vitamin deficiencies, or simple aging.

Bizarre Symptoms of Dizziness

Less common symptoms of "dizziness" include complaints such as "the world is always tilted," or, "my vision goes dark." Although such complaints are typical of neurologic disorders, such complaints are occasionally expressed by those with vestibular problems. When a person experiences vertigo, this new experience for the patient is upsetting emotionally, often causing the patient to feel as if he or she is having a medical emergency. It is not uncommon for a patient with vestibular disorder to say he or she "passed out," which often just means the patient fell down due to the vertigo. It should be realized, however, that true medical emergencies can also cause vertigo mimicking that caused by inner ear disorders. The author has witnessed vestibular-looking nystagmus in patients just before they passed out from nonvestibular causes. One memorable patient presenting to our otolaryngology office with what was assumed to be typical "vestibular" nystagmus and severe vertigo of recent onset was admitted to the hospital and found to have a large nonacoustic tumor. All descriptions of bizarre dizziness should be considered serious until proven otherwise.

Problems with a sense of body position can also occur in the **somatosensory proprioceptive**, and **visual** systems. It should be noted that there are also portions of the vestibular system involved in muscle responses to position changes such as the **vestibulospinal** and **vestibulocolic** tracts, which send motor signals to the arms and legs or neck, respectively.

Miscellaneous Terms
(Woozy, Heavy Head, Not Myself)

Although the terms "woozy," "heavy headed," or "not myself" are sometimes used by patients who simply feel ill and have no feelings of motion or lightheadedness, these terms are sometimes used by patients who do have vestibular disorders such as BPPV or some other "**uncompensated vestibulopathy**." Asking, "does quickly moving your head bring these symptoms on?" helps to indicate a true vestibular disorder.

Help for Those with Dizziness

Although dizziness is one of the most common complaints, it is rarely a permanent condition. However, treatment must be diligently sought because there are obstacles to overcome in its correction. As can be imagined from the above discussion, **it is difficult for the patient to obtain a correct diagnosis**. There are two main reasons for this. First, dizziness is common in a wide variety of disorders, and second, health practitioners often seek to first rule out life-threatening disorders by ordering CT scans or other more lengthy tests. Patients often become discouraged at about the third doctor visit when they are still told that there is not yet a definitive diagnosis. Notwithstanding these obstacles, assuming there is not a rapidly deteriorating medical condition, patients do not have to live with constant dizziness. For example, the body's tremendous compensatory mechanisms will eliminate vertigo due to most inner ear causes in time if the person moves enough, which allows the brain to "compensate" for the disorder. If the level of activity is low, exercises specifically intended for compensation may be required (vestibular rehabilitation). If the inner ear problem is chronic, otolaryngologic intervention can ultimately eliminate the vertigo in most if not all cases. If a person's "dizziness" is not due to "inner ear" disorder, but is due to other "internal medicine" disorders such as diabetes, proper medical intervention ultimately will result in a permanent solution to these feelings in many cases. Too often, a comment is heard from patients suffering from dizziness is that the condition is just part of getting older. Whereas this may be true of *imbalance*, it is not usually the case with dizziness. In our practice, many patients are seen who have been suffering for years with an **uncompensated vestibulopathy**, usually starting with a severe, sudden onset of vertigo due to inner ear disorder, but now several years afterward are still having a mild vertigo when the head or body is moving. After appropriate exercises or other therapies, such patients are often surprised that the dizziness has been eliminated.

In summary, dizziness is a term too commonly used for a variety of symptoms having numerous possible etiologies. Although diagnoses often take time to achieve due to clinicians having to prioritize the examination toward life-threatening causes, most cases of dizziness are eventually properly diagnosed and successfully rehabilitated.

CHAPTER 5

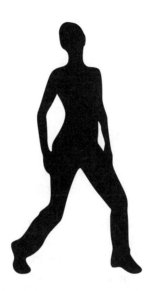

The Falls Clinic and Examination

The term "Falls Clinic" is used in this book to refer to a comprehensive clinic in which both diagnostic and rehabilitative issues are addressed. Unfortunately, the term is being rather loosely utilized in some locations to give the impression of a comprehensive clinic, when in reality some of these offer only a limited range of services, being primarily vestibular clinics combined with vestibular rehabilitation. Because of the wide variety of medical causes of falls, a true falls clinic should address multiple body systems as well as provide a number of rehabilitation options. At the time of this writing, relatively few comprehensive "Falls Clinics" exist.

Description of the Falls Clinic

To begin, we take a sample journey of a "typical" patient at a visit to the Falls Clinic. A typical case visiting the Falls Clinic is described in Case 1 of Chapter 8, which gives a narrative description. The clinic described is the Falls Prevention Clinic at Henry Ford Hospital, Detroit, Michigan. This hypothetical patient described is a composite of many similar patients.

Why We Do What We Do

The patient undergoes two visits, which usually include consultation by an audiologist, internal medicine specialist, and physical therapist. Included are "falls history," describing the number and type of falls, vestibular and balance functioning testing, as well as testing of all other body systems capable of causing falls. At the end of the second visit, a counseling session by the team occurs in which the information obtained is related to the patient and family as well as recommendations for physical therapy or other interventions such as modification of lifestyle or living environment. Often the patient and family, when presented with the findings and particular falls risk situations, will come up with their own solutions.

Multispecialty Format

The multispecialty nature of the clinic accomplishes several things. In terms of convenience, the patient obtains a thorough evaluation at a single location. More importantly, the clinicians have the opportunity of conferring with one another which helps put the various individual problems into perspective. Without the group model, the following would have likely happened with the sample patient. She most likely would have been referred to one of several specialists by her primary doctor. If this had been an otolaryngologist, chances are high her vesibulopathy would have been identified but admittedly her orthostatic hypotension would probably not have been. On the other hand, if she had visited a cardiologist first, the entire problem might have been attributed to her orthostatic hypotension. A common problem is that specialists tend to attribute falling problems to the disorder discovered only within their own specialty area. The comment "multifactorial causes" seems to be overutilized in place of sending the patient to yet another specialist. Only by seeing the patient within the framework of a group evaluation would a perspective be achieved regarding the "main cause" of falls. Such a "runaround" scenario is especially likely to happen with older patients who often have multiple minor disorders. When attempting to find the "main cause," it is helpful to consider the nature and circumstances of the falls in the context of a multispecialty clinic. For example, if a patient has both orthostatic hypotension as well as vestibulopathy, but falls mainly when there is inadequate lighting, then the vestibulopathy is more likely the main cause.

The contribution of the **internal medicine** specialist to our clinic is invaluable because of the many cardiovascular, general medical, and medication issues contributing to falls. This particular specialty is well suited to discovering and reviewing these issues with the patient. This is not to say that certain other specialties could not accomplish this task at an acceptable level. It is likely that neurologists would also be valuable team members.

Having the **physical therapist** on site during the evaluation is also a very useful component in helping the falls clinic achieve a "one-stop shopping" or "executive physical" format. Not only does the physical therapist evaluate the need and potential of strength and gait training, but the assessment of the environment, personal habits, and suggestions for safety equipment for the home are invaluable. It is also the physical therapist who is best suited to recommend walking aids such as canes and walkers.

Vestibular Rehabilitation

In the sample case referred to (see Case 1 in Chapter 8), the main correctable cause of falling was determined to be the nonspecific "**uncompensated vestibulopathy**," often due to previous **vestibular neuritis**. The recent interest in treatment of this disorder through vestibular rehabilitation techniques has significantly helped reduce symptoms of imbalance in many people. Second only to benign positional vertigo in occurrence, we find uncompensated vestibulopathy the cause of a significant percentage of patients presenting to the Falls Clinic. We find that, in addition to standard balance function test (VNG, rotational chair, posturography) the use of the "head shake" test or other high-speed head rotation test is indispensable in identifying uncompensated vestibulopathies. Rotational chair and caloric testing using VNG test at too slow head rotation speeds to determine whether complete compensation has occurred. Our definition of nonspecific "uncompensated vestibulopathy" is abnormality on high-speed rotational tests along with symptoms that correlate with a vestibular disorder. Uncompensated vestibulopathy, assumed to be due to previous peripheral vestibular insult, can be caused by a wide variety of initial disorders, such as vestibular neuronitis, vestibular labrynthitis, or other cause, in which permanent or temporary damage has occurred at one of the vestibular end organs. Regardless of the cause, patients usually feel that since the initial symptoms began they are "just a little off, especially with head movement." This condition has not completely compensated because the patient has not been active enough or moved the head often or quickly enough for the brain to readjust to the imbalance of the vestibular output of the two ears. What is needed for the patient to finally compensate, are exercises that integrate the eyes with the vestibular system (**vestibular-ocular reflex**). Such "vestibular rehabilitation exercises" involve head movements of various types while focusing the eyes on visual targets. Courses are available for training in the latest techniques of vestibular rehabilitation. Months of therapy, which can sometimes be self-directed, are typically required to completely accomplish the rehabilitation. Fortunately, exercises are painless, although the patient will often feel greater dizziness in the initial stages of the exercises. If self-directed exercises are inadequate for complete compensation, the therapist can direct the patient over a period of weeks.

Finding the "Main Cause" of Falls

Although postural hypotension and uncompensated vestibulopathy represent some of the more common ones, other common disorders present to the Falls Clinic in various combinations, including **peripheral neuropathy, medication effects, benign paroxysmal positional vertigo, cardiovascular problems, migraine and weakness in the lower extremities compared to body**

mass. Most aging patients will have more than one disorder; however, there is usually one disorder that can be considered the "**main cause**." After discovering all of the falls risk factors, it should be the goal of the evaluation to determine this main cause of falls. Stating that the cause of the patient's falls is "multifactorial" is often an excuse for not being able to determine a main cause of the patient's falls. Observing the patient in various real-world balance situations will help the examiner determine the main mechanisms of falling. Having the patient describe the most recent falls also helps with this determination.

Behavior Modification

Behavior modification is an area in which most audiologists are not well trained; however, modifying behavior is a large part of what makes the Falls Clinic successful. In Mary's case, a lifelong penchant for rushing is now becoming a liability to her. Some would argue that the exercise she has obtained by being high strung has helped to contribute to her strength at this point in her life. Some may wonder if trying to slow her down is really in her best interests. In reality, she does need to modify some of her behaviors if she wants to prevent more falls because it was determined during the questioning that rushing was contributing to her falls. The reader is referred to the section in Chapter 6 on behavior modification. In addition, safe exercise such as holding onto a shopping cart for support would increase her strength, further reducing falls and injury risk. The "SafeWalk" techniques described in Chapter 6 also are helpful in modifying behaviors in that they help replace old habits with new ones aimed at slower, more deliberate ambulation.

Components of the Falls Clinic

Table 5–1 shows the components of the clinic through which each patient passes. Patients typically make two visits to the clinic. At the first visit, termed "Balance Function Test," the patient receives either a full vestibular test battery or, if the history is not suggestive of vestibular involvement, a "vestibular screening." More about who receives only the screening is discussed later. At the second visit,

Table 5–1. Components of the Falls Clinic

Before the Visit

Referral received

Patient's records reviewed

Patient is scheduled for vestibular testing

Visit One

History of falls and balance

Examination of vestibular systems

Visit Two

History of falls circumstances

Examination of nonvestibular systems

Physical therapy examination

Summary meeting

Follow-Up Phone Call

Patient contacted by phone or letter

the patient receives assessment of the nonvestibular body systems, an assessment for physical therapy candidacy, as well an examination of other "extrinsic" factors. These include the patient's environment, living conditions, and social interactions.

The second visit is usually attended by a physical therapist, as well as an internal medicine specialist. At the end of the second visit, the patient is counseled by the examiners in a group session including the patient's family or caregivers if possible. At the counseling, not only are results presented, but strategies and plans are discussed for preventing future falls. A full written report is furnished to the patient at the end of the visit or at least a written list of recommendations to be followed by a written report. The patient receives a follow-up phone call or letter inquiring about the patient's current falls, if any. The patient reports on the number of falls since the visit so that it may be determined whether or not the recommendations are working.

Following is a description of what occurs in each of the Falls Clinic visits.

First Visit

Referral

Generally, patients have been referred by a physician. If not, a written physician referral is obtained. Records of these referring visits are obtained or a detailed medical history is related by the patient if obtaining the actual records is not possible.

History

The case history (see Appendix B for sample forms) should include general medical conditions possibly contributing to falls, present symptoms, and circumstances surrounding falls during the past 6 months. A portion of this history may be filled out by the patient in the waiting room. As shown, important information regarding the number of falls is obtained. As there is always the risk of dishonesty on this question we have found that the following measures are helpful. Have the other two team members, the physical therapist and internal medicine specialist, also ask the question regarding number of falls. Very often, the patient will confide in one of the three examiners but deny falls to the other two. As with the sample patient (see Case 1 in Chapter 8), it is striking to see the high number of falls that patients coming to the Falls Clinic experience. The notion that there is "one big fall" that "grandma" will have and break her hip is soon dispelled by asking patients presenting to the clinic how many times they have fallen, although obtaining the truth from patients is often difficult. The fear of losing more independence is high motivation for patients not to be completely truthful about the number of falls they have had. When asking whether or not falls occur, we have found it more effective to simply ask **how many** falls have occurred in the past 6 months instead of just asking, "have you fallen?" the answer to which is usually "no." By asking "how many times have you fallen?" the patient more easily assumes that falling is occurring many times in the typical patient, which encourages more truthfulness. Still, the answer may be an underestimate of the actual number of falls but at least a positive answer will confirm that falls are indeed occurring. Previous studies have indicated that most falls do not result in injury, but it is undeniable ongoing falls will eventually result in injury. Sometimes the patient, while alone with the examiner, will admit to falls and other unfortunate behavior such as climbing stairs more often on the knees, but add "please don't tell my daughter that."

Examination of Vestibular Systems

During the first visit, patients either undergo a full vestibular test battery, including VNG/ENG, rotational chair, and computerized dynamic platform posturography, or if appropriate, more limited testing (vestibular screening). The term screening is really a misnomer in that screening usually refers to the testing of large numbers of asymptomatic individuals. In our case, limited vestibular testing is warranted in some patients who do not have signs or complaints of vestibular symptoms, but who are falling. Such "screening" is probably adequate if there is little chance in the referring otolaryngologist's mind of there being a vestibular disorder. These "screenings" should properly be referred to as "**preliminary vestibular testing**." This preliminary vestibular testing does pick up a large number of previously unsuspected vestibulopathies. This testing consists of observing for nystagmus using video goggles with vision denied as well as performing other "bedside" vestibular tests to be described. Deciding who gets only the limited testing is an important issue. Erring on the side of the full testing would probably be wise as currently there is not adequate research data to show the effectiveness of only the limited protocol. The limited testing should therefore be used only for those for whom there are no complaints of dizziness or vertigo, nor significant past history of such. If there is any suspicion of vestibular problems, the full testing should be carried out, consisting of a minimum of full VNG, posturography, and rotational chair. Testing should also include other tests such as VEMP (**vestibular evoked myogenic potentials**) for determining the function of the vestibule colic reflex (reflex aiding the head's stability upon the neck), **high-speed head rotation**, and **fistula testing** (determining a leak of inner ear fluid) if warranted. Because many patients, such as those with BPPV, do not have typical complaints of frank "vertigo," everyone should have at least the vestibular "screening," even if the patient says there is no dizziness or vertigo. Patients who say "I am not dizzy, just a little off" are often found to have BPPV or uncompensated vestibulopathy. It should be noted that the term "screening" is frowned upon by insurance carriers when it comes to audiologic tests because it implies that many normals will be "screened" to discover future candidates for testing such as potential hearing aid patients. In this case, "screening" is not the most appropriate term for the limited vestibular testing suggested here; rather, a minimum number of appropriate tests are being chosen for the patient who is not suspected of having vestibulopathy.

Preliminary Vestibular Testing ("Screening")

Table 5-2 shows the tests employed in the Vestibular Screening (also termed "preliminary vestibular testing"). Failure on any portion of the examination indicates the need for the complete Balance Function Testing just described.

Table 5–2. Preliminary Vestibular Testing (Screening)*

History
Hearing test (any unexplained loss or asymmetric loss that has not been "worked up" for acoustic neuroma)
Nystagmus under video goggles (vision denied)   • Spontaneous   • Gaze-evoked nystagmus (vision denied)   • High-frequency head shake
Hallpike
Bedside balance tests: Romberg, Fukuda, Head thrust, Standing on foam (Gans Sensory Organization Performance Test)

*Failure on any one, including history consistent with vestibular disorder, constitutes failure of the screening and necessitates full vestibular testing)

Nystagmus

Because nystagmus of the "peripheral type" (see description below) is the hallmark of a vestibular disorder, it is important to carefully check for this using video goggles with vision denied so that the central visual system does not suppress the nystagmus. Peripheral vestibular type nystagmus is worse or only present with eyes covered (in the dark), is enhanced when looking in the direction of the fast phase (Alexander's law), and is usually enhanced or discovered after shaking the head (again with eyes covered). Our screening protocol, after taking the history, is to have the patient stare straight ahead while wearing the video goggles with eyes covered. Spontaneous nystagmus is observed. If present, the patient is asked to gaze approximately 30 degrees to the right for several seconds, then 30 degrees to the left, again for several seconds. Looking too far to the side may induce a normal "endpoint nystagmus." This would be distinguished because it would occur on either side; therefore, if nystagmus is only observed on one side, or is markedly greater on one side than the other, the nystagmus is probably significant and not just representing "endpoint nystagmus." Again, do not have the patient gaze too far to either side. With experience using the 30-degree targets used on ENG or VNG, the examiner will become proficient in recognizing when the patient is gazing too far. Another method is to have the patient look with eyes open at the 30-degree mark, then pretend to be looking at the same mark when the eyes are immediately covered.

Head Shake Test

After the spontaneous and gaze nystagmus have been observed, **head shake** testing is performed. This is accomplished by having the patient, while wearing the goggles (vision denied), shake the head briskly back and forth for 20 to 30 seconds. The patient then stops, and with eyes opened, any nystagmus is observed. The presence of more than two definite beats indicates an abnormal test. The head shake test has been studied for several years and has received both good and bad reviews. Most criticism, however, is regarding whether the test is sensitive enough or specific enough to a particular type of ear disorder. These issues, however, do not detract from its usefulness as a screening measure as the purpose of screening is to simply identify any vestibular problem. Head shake-induced nystagmus is present in some normal patients (reportedly as high as 20%) as well as in various neurologic disorders. Head-shake-induced nystagmus is, therefore, a rather sensitive test, but not very specific as to type of disorder. Its tendency is to overrefer for vestibular disorder. Therefore, an abnormal result on the test should be considered ample grounds for further vestibular testing. Passing the test, however, should also not be considered adequate evidence of the lack of a vestibular problem. In our experience, the head shake test, combined with the history, is a very useful tool and is used currently by many expert clinicians as one of the most effective indicators of a vestibular disorder (see Hain, Fetter, & Zee [1987] and Wei, Hain, & Proctor [1989]).

Hallpike

The Dix-Hallpike test, familiar to most audiologists as well as many other health care providers, is explained in detail in several texts. Some modifications also exist to suit the needs of various types of physical limitations in patients. The reader is referred to Viirre, Purcell, and Baloh (2005).

Because there is controversy regarding some issues when applying the standard technique, we focus our insights into some of these issues, recognizing that any variation in the classic procedure has certain pros and cons. For example, the original technique did not advocate the use of video goggles (they did not exist at the time). Use of video goggles either with vision denied or not denied holds the advantage of being able to record eye movements for further future review. A disadvantage is simply that it is sometimes difficult to hold the patient securely and manage the position of the goggles at the same time. Also, if the patient focuses the eyes on some portion of the goggles this may reduce or fixate the response completely. Having the eyes covered (vision denied) also has the same fixation possibility if there is any light leakage into the goggles. It is argued that having vision denied is not necessary because the eye movement response seen in patients with positive Hallpike is impossible to inhibit. This is usually the case; however, the author has tested a patient recently whose Hallpike first was negative but immediately afterward was positive when using goggles with vision denied. This may have an alternative explanation, however.

It has been suggested that the Hallpike be tried twice because sometimes it will be positive the second time especially if the person lays on the side after the first trial which may allow for particles to collect (Viirre, Purcell, & Baloh 2005).

Some authors are careful to point out that, as the Hallpike response is a fatigable one, the patient should not be moved more than absolutely necessary before the Hallpike is performed. We see nothing wrong with this philosophy and try to perform the Hallpike as early in the exam as possible. We also feel that the fatigability factor can also inhibit the head shake test. On the other hand, having the patient shake the head too early in the exam may cause nystagmus that may not fatigue for several minutes, thus interfering with the spontaneous or positional tests. We therefore modify our order in accordance with what we may expect to find. It is not known exactly how much of an effect modifying the order of VNG subtests has on the various outcomes. It is likely that this is not a very important issue in most cases.

Other authors have advocated alternative procedures for performing the Hallpike test to accommodate various body limitations for performing the standard maneuver. We see nothing wrong with such modifications, assuming that they all have the result of the head ending up in the same general position.

Bedside Vestibular Tests

Next, the "bedside" tests for vestibular disorder are performed. These informal tests are important in the screening process because standard VNG/ENG and rotational chair do not emphasize the vestibulo-spinal tract or other accessory vestibular pathways. Although posturography does give some indication of the utilization of the vestibule-spinal tracts, other testing is also indicated in order to assess the entire vestibular system. Vestibular evoked myogenic potentials (VEMP) is a test that can be used to assess the vestibulo-colic reflex, which is a subsystem of the vestibulospinal tract. However, some of the less technical tests are also useful for assessing the overall vestibular system. The bedside tests we employ are the **Romberg** test (Khasnis & Gokula, 2003), **Fukuda** test (Fukuda, 1959, 1984), **"head thrust"** test (Halmagyi & Curthoys, 1988; Herdman, 2004) and the Gans Sensory Organization Performance Test (American Institute of Balance, Seminole, Florida). These tests are illustrated in Figures 5-1, 5-2, and 5-3.

Romberg Test

The patient stands with feet together and arms hanging at the sides. The examiner stands close facing the patient so that if a fall occurs it can be stopped by the examiner. The examiner observes the patient for 1 minute (according to the original version of the test) with eyes open and then with eyes closed. A "positive Romberg" or "Romberg's sign" occurs only when the patient can stand with eyes

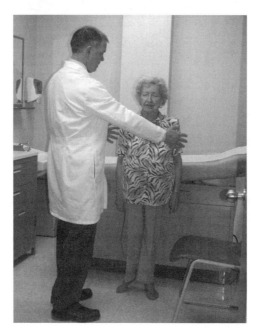

Figure 5–1. Romberg test. Patient attempts to keep balance with eyes closed. A near fall is a positive test. The examiner should have something behind the patient such as a chair in case of a fall backward.

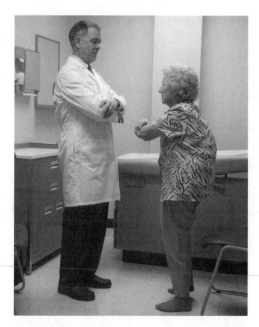

Figure 5–2.   Fukuda test. Patient marches with eyes closed while attempting to not turn to the right or left. A turn greater than 30 degrees or near fall is considered abnormal.

open but not with eyes closed. The test is thought by many to be most useful for detecting sensory ataxia; however, patients having vestibular disorders will often fall toward the abnormal side or backward. Patients with other central problems such as cerebellar disorders will often fall with eyes open as well as closed. Having the patient place one foot forward as in taking a step makes this test more difficult and more sensitive ("tandem Romberg" or "sharpened Romberg").

Fukuda Test

The patient with eyes closed and arms stretched out or folded, attempts to march briskly in place for approximately 30 steps. A turn off-center 30 degrees or less is considered normal. Patients with vestibular disorder will usually slump or fall to the abnormal side, or

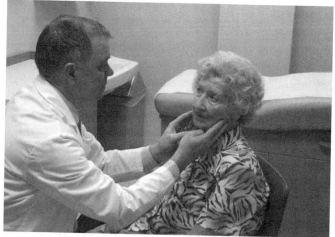

A.

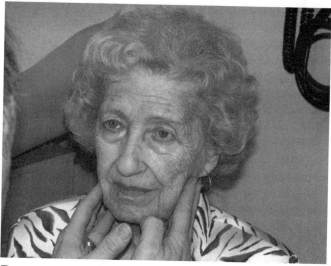

B.

Figure 5–3. Head thrust test. The examiner tells the patient that at any moment, the head will be moved rapidly to the center. The patient is asked to keep the eyes focused on the examiner's nose at all times and to keep the neck loose (**A**). The head is moved rapidly to the midline (**B**). If the eyes continue past the midline, this is a positive (abnormal) test, indicating vestibulopathy that is usually on the side the head is moving toward. *Note*: One very small compensatory saccade is not abnormal.

occasionally wander away from the bad side without any slumping or falling. It has been pointed out that patients with somatosensory disorders, tonic neck reflexes, faulty tonic lumbar reflexes, or kinesthetic disorders also will have a positive Fukuda (Fukushima & Hinoki, 1985; Gordon, Fletcher, Jones, & Block, 1995a, 1995b).

Head Thrust Test

The patient is grasped gently by the head and told to focus the eyes on a target, usually the tester's nose. The patient is told that you are going to gently but quickly turn his head while observing the eyes. Starting with the head slightly to the side, the patient's head is briskly turned to the center position. The patient's eyes should stay focused on the target. If the eyes continue past the target and then quickly move back using a "corrective saccade," it indicates a reduced vestibular response on the side the head was turned toward. The procedure is repeated with a head turn in the other direction. Sometimes a normal patient will exhibit a very small single corrective saccade but this should happen with head turns in either direction and should be symmetric. With a vestibular lesion, the eyes, instead of remaining on the target, will continue on past center, and then return to center by the definite corrective saccade (see Minor et al., 2001).

Gans Sensory Organization Performance Test

The patient's ability to stand is compared for the conditions—thick foam with eyes open or closed, standing on the floor (traditional Romberg and sharpened Romberg) as well as marching (Fukuda test). Key to the differentiation is the patient's performance on the foam, where falling with eyes closed signifies vestibular, whereas falling with eyes open indicates central pathology (American Institute of Balance, Seminole, Florida).

Audiogram

A hearing test is important for any patient exhibiting dizziness, imbalance, or vertigo. Although most vestibular disorders do not exhibit hearing loss, the more serious ones often do. Any unexpected or unexplained hearing loss is grounds for failing the vestibular screening. Asymmetric losses are especially suspect for suggesting vestibular disorder as are severe bilateral losses, in which case a bilateral reduced vestibular response on caloric testing may be suspected. Progressive losses are also suspect for indicating vestibular disorder. Hearing loss can also occasionally indicate central nervous system pathology. In short, any hearing loss that is not explained by age alone or previous workup by an ENT doctor, should render the screening test "abnormal," thereby requiring the full vestibular testing.

Full Vestibular Evaluation

The following sections briefly describe the tests utilized in a comprehensive vestibular evaluation. Greater details on these tests can be found in several excellent current texts. Evaluating the entire vestibular system is difficult because of the complexity of the ancillary subsystems including vestibulospinal, cervical vestibular, and others. To test these portions of the vestibular system, a combination of bedside tests (see previous section) and more formal tests such as VEMP (vestibular evoked myogenic potentials) which tests the vestibulocolic reflex, may be employed. Establishing normal function of the "inner ear" vestibular system, which is more often the offending subsystem, is less challenging; however, ENG or VNG alone is not adequate to establish normal function of the labyrinthine vestibular system. Many vestibular abnormalities are detected only by using test frequencies higher than that simulated by ENG or VNG caloric irrigations. Caloric irrigations simulate only very slow head rotation speeds. Testing at higher speeds than are available even on most rotary chairs is necessary to simulate the faster head movements typical of everyday life. Using the "head shake test" with video goggles is one way to accomplish higher head speed testing. The VAT (vestibular autorotation test) is an electronic version of this concept.

VNG/ENG

Electronystagmography (ENG), and its counterpart VNG, which uses video goggles instead of electrodes to measure eye movements, constitute the "work horses" of vestibular testing. These two tests accomplish the same thing, namely, measuring eye movements under various stimulus conditions. Abnormal eye movements, particularly "nystagmus," are the hallmark of a vestibular disorder. ENG/VNG is also useful for determining oculomotor function.

Eye Movements

Eye movements are important to vestibular as well as oculomotor assessment for several reasons. Involuntary eye jerks or "nystagmus" is an indication of either central nervous system or vestibular system abnormality. Nystagmus is designated as being either "right beating" or "left beating" to signify which direction the fast phase is directed toward. For example, "right beating" nystagmus would be eyes jerking with a fast component toward the right, followed by a slower return movement to the left. Vestibular nystagmus is produced due to the "vestibulo-ocular reflex," a crossed reflex arc. When the right ear is stimulated, either by warm temperature or movement toward it, nerve impulses are transmitted to the opposite side of the head, activating the left eye's lateral rectus and the right eye's medial rectus muscle, causing the eyes to move to the left. At the same time, the opposite muscles are inhibited due to destimulation of the left ear (fluid moving away from the left ear), which causes the opposite muscles to relax. The central nervous system finally snaps the eyes quickly back to center position. Thus, the slow component is produced by the vestibular system, whereas the fast component is produced by the central nervous system. Pathologic forms of vestibular nystagmus occurs when there is an imbalance somewhere in the pathway. This may occur with an "irritative lesion," one that stimulates one of the ears artificially, or an "ablative lesion," one in which there is a reduction in function of one of the ears. This has been a somewhat oversimplified explanation of nystagmus. Detailed discussions of nystagmus are found in various textbooks that are easily obtainable.

Central nervous system nystagmus is rare and has particular identifying characteristics. In contrast, peripheral vestibular nystagmus is quite common and has its own set of identifying characteristics. Table 2–2 in Chapter 2 contrasts central versus peripheral vestibular nystagmus. Peripheral vestibular nystagmus has the characteristic of being greater with eyes closed (or only discernible to the tester when the patient's eyes are closed). Also, peripheral nystagmus is often greater when gazing with eyes closed toward the direction of the fast component (Alexander's law). In addition, peripheral nystagmus does not change direction within a single head position. In contrast, central nervous system nystagmus is often greater with eyes open (or at least no less with eyes open than closed), only present with eyes open, present only when gazing off center with eyes open, or is vertical in nature. Other types of eye movements are also considered central signs such as "disconjugate" eye movements (eyes not moving in synchrony).

Absence of nystagmus, or reduced amplitude nystagmus, is also a sign of vestibular disorder. When an ear is warmed or cooled individually by an air or water irrigation, nystagmus should be elicited beating either toward or away from the side irrigated, respectively. For example, following the acronym "COWS" (cold opposite, warm same), a cool irrigation to the normal right ear would produce left-beating nystagmus; whereas, a warm irrigation to the normal left ear would produce left-beating nystagmus. Another example of nystagmus being normal in a test would be in rotational chair (see next section). When a patient undergoes this test, he or she is seated in a dark chamber in a chair that can rotate in either direction. Rotation toward the patient's right should produce right-beating nystagmus, whereas rotation to the left produces left-beating nystagmus. This happens because fluid in the right horizontal semicircular canal is moving toward the sensory cells in the "ampulla" stimulating that ear, whereas fluid in the opposite (left) ear's horizontal canal is moving away from the ampulla, thus inhibiting it.

Tests Within the ENG/VNG Battery

Oculomotor: These are eye tests aimed at assessing voluntary or reflexive eye movements using a visual target.

1. The "**saccade**" test evaluates very rapid eye movements by determining the ability to move the eyes to a dot suddenly appearing at random locations. Abnormalities include increased latency of the eyes relative to the target or decreased accuracy or velocity compared to similar aged

norms. The pattern for normal results are "square waves" in which velocity, latency, and accuracy are appropriate for the age of the patient.

2. The "**pendular tracking**" test, also called smooth pursuit, tests the ability of the eyes to follow a smoothly moving target at various speeds.

3. The "**optokinetic test**" (OKN or OPK) assesses the eye movements in response to a moving visual surround or moving background occupying the entire visual field. Reflexive nystagmus occurs and is said to be caused by central mechanisms, the "optokinetic system." Abnormality is an asymmetric response between clockwise and counterclockwise motion and may be caused by either central or vestibular abnormality.

Vestibular system tests:

1. **Nystagmus testing**—Using either the electrodes at the sides of the eyes already mentioned or video goggles, the presence of abnormal nystagmus is determined both with eyes open or closed. The conditions utilized include

   a. *Spontaneous*—Nystagmus is determined with the patient sitting starring at a target (visual suppression) as well as with eyes closed or covered using video goggles. The presence of nystagmus signifies either central or peripheral vestibular abnormality as previously discussed (see Table 2-2 in Chapter 2). There are also cases of congenital nystagmus, which is usually known to the patient.

   b. *Gaze test*—Nystagmus is observed with the patient gazing 30 degrees to the right, left, up, or down. Nystagmus to left or right gaze can be a central or peripheral sign. A spontaneous nystagmus at central gaze (eyes closed) that is enhanced when gazing in the direction of the fast phase, is usually a peripheral sign (Alexander's law). Gaze nystagmus with eyes open can be a central sign but is also normal in some if mild and present in both directions ("endpoint nystagmus").

   c. *Positional*—Nystagmus is searched for when the patient is lying supine or with head or body to the right or left, as well as head hanging as in the Hallipike test previously described. Positional nystagmus is commonly associated with benign positional vertigo, as in horizontal canal **canalythiasis, or cupulolythiasis** for which repositioning maneuvers are commonly performed. Positional nystamgus, if changing position in a single position, is associated with a central disorder.

Rotational Chair Testing

Testing for vestibular function using a pivoting chair has been in use for many years. Nystagmus is produced in normals in the direction of the spinning; thus, a spin to the patient's right causes a right-beating nystagmus as long as the motion is accelerating. Once a constant speed is attained then nystagmus will begin to stop because the semicircular canal system is sensitive to acceleration or deceleration only and not constant velocity. Although both ears are stimulated by spinning, isolation of one of the ears for evaluation is not possible; nonetheless, some useful information may be obtained by such testing. In earlier days, physicians would spin a patient in a chair a number of times and then stop the patient abruptly. The length of time the nystagmus lasted was compared for a clockwise or counterclockwise spin. Establishing a rough symmetry of the responses in either direction was evidence of a balanced response of the right and left vestibular systems. Amount of nystagmus observed was also useful. Patients in whom a bilateral reduced vestibular response was present would exhibit a smaller amount of eye beating or none at all in either direction of spin. An asymmetry however, simply meant that one of the ears was either functioning at a reduced or hyperactive level. It was impossible to tell which ear was the offending side.

Modern Rotational Chairs

Modern rotational chairs perform the same basic assessment as the simple pivot chairs, only now normative data may be utilized and greater accuracy is attained. Similar to the olden days, the offending side is still difficult to pinpoint; however, by use of other accompanying tests such as VNG, the abnormal side can usually be established.

Advantages of Rotational Chair Testing

Although not as sensitive as VNG/ENG, the rotational chair test is good when irrigations are hard to perform, when irrigations may not be accurate as in a perforation, and so forth, or when a child is afraid of irrigations (the child can do rotational chair on Mom's lap), or as a double check of the VNG/ENG findings.

Disadvantages of Rotational Chair Testing

Although rotational chair testing cannot technically localize left versus right ear disorder, sometimes it is obvious (more on this below). Another limitation is that, just as in VNG, the stimulus simulates a very slow head rotation, much slower than typical movements of real life. Although rotational chair testing uses a slightly higher speed than simulated by the VNG irrigations, it is still very slow and misses some **uncompensated vestibulopathies** that the higher speed tests such as head shake and VAT can determine (more on this in the "symmetry" section below).

Abnormal Findings

A "**phase lead**" is one of the hallmarks of a vestibular disorder on the rotational chair test. Phase refers to the position of the eyes in relation to the moving chair. Why do abnormal phase leads occur in a vestibular disorder? One of the vestibular system's functions is to determine the velocity of head rotation and store this information. This function which occurs in the brainstem is called **velocity storage**. In vestibular disorders there is a loss of velocity storage, perhaps through lack of input. When this occurs, there is inaccuracy, in the dark, in the ability of the eyes to move in response to the movement of the chair; that is, the vestibular-ocular reflex is inaccurate and typically results in a phase lead of the eye's movement compared to the chair's movement. Phase leads therefore represent vestibular disorder due to loss of velocity storage. **Phase lags**, which are actually not "lags," but lower than normal phase leads, are usually due to test error, but can on occasion be a central sign. To summarize phase findings, higher than normal phase leads mean vestibular abnormality, whereas lower than normal phase leads usually just mean calibration error but can occasionally mean central abnormality.

Symmetry refers to the balance of nystagmus that should be achieved with rotation in either direction. An asymmetric response means that one ear is weak or the other is hyperreactive to movement. The question is, "Can we ascertain which 'ear' has the problem?" The answer to this is, "no, not with certainty." Usually, however, an apparent weakness to one side usually indicates a weakness in that ear, although it is possible that the opposite ear is hyperreactive (as in Ménière's disease at certain stages of the disorder). So what good is the symmetry measure? Asymmetry is another hallmark of a vestibular disorder. If there *is* symmetry, however, there can still be a vestibular disorder but the disorder is usually long standing (chronic or "compensated") meaning that if the disorder is long standing, the central mechanism will eventually readjust and the asymmetry disappears. But asymmetry, if present, is usually a clear sign of vestibular disease. To summarize phase lead findings, phase leads with symmetry signify chronic vestibular disorder, whereas phase leads with asymmetry signify acute disorder.

Gain refers to the strength or degree of nystagmus produced by the chair rotation. In bilateral weakness there will be little or no nystagmus and therefore low gain values. But there needs to be only one good ear to show adequate gain, so low gain values must mean that both ears are below par. The other more common possibility with low gains is that of test error, usually that the patient is not performing the alerting task well enough or does not have his or her eyes open enough. Low gains, if due to test error and not bilateral weakness, render the phase and symmetry data uninterpretable at that frequency.

To summarize gain findings, low gains usually mean test error rendering the data at that frequency uninterpretable, or low gains can also mean a bilateral weakness, which should also show up on calorics. Higher than normal gains do not usually mean anything abnormal.

Rotational chair testing provides a welcome addition to the vestibular test battery. There are many instances in which caloric responses cannot be adequately obtained. Ear canals of smaller size or unusual or asymmetric shape often makes irrigation by either air or water difficult and unreliable. A false positive for unilateral or bilateral weakness can be obtained quite often in ENG or VNG; therefore, the second independent test provided by rotational chair testing is often important. Newer concepts in rotational chair testing are beginning to emerge. "Off-axis" chairs, for example, undoubtedly will show advantages in determining more specific information. Higher speed chairs are also beginning to become available, which will more closely approximate head speeds encountered in everyday living and thereby help determine whether a vestibular lesion has indeed been completely compensated. Until high-speed chairs are more readily available, less expensive measures such as the head shake test or the VAT test will be expected to be more extensively utilized to rule out uncompensated vestibulopathy at higher head speed rotations.

Posturography

Computerized dynamic platform posturography (CDPP) is another useful device for both diagnostic as well as rehabilitative purposes. As with rotational chair testing, CDPP has been available in a "low tech" form for many years. The older "foam and dome" test requires the patient to stand on foam, thus eliminating the somatosensory balance sense. At the same time, a dome of some sort would be placed over the patient's head blocking the vision. The patient is then left with only the vestibular system for balance. Inability to stand on the foam with either the dome covering the eyes or simply with the eyes closed would identify a vestibular problem. A formalized version of this test has been introduced, the Gans Sensory Organization Performance Test, in which a piece of thick foam is used on which the patient's ability to stand with eyes open or closed is determined and compared to other conditions such as the Romberg and Fukuda tests (see above). Inability to stand on the foam with eyes open generally signals a problem of a greater extent than peripheral vestibular such as neurologic or global disorder. A similar test using this concept is the CTSIB (El-Kashlan et al., 1998; Wrisley & Whitney, 2004;) in which a computerized force plate is utilized.

In computerized dynamic platform posturography (CDPP) (Neurocom, Portland, OR), the patient stands on a computer-monitored force plate that detects the patient's center of gravity, direction of tilt of the body, as well as other aspects of balance. The patient's balance is measured under different conditions such as standing with eyes open or closed, having to balance on a hinged platform, standing while the platform is fixed but the visual surround is moving, and so forth. These conditions isolate the somatosensory, vestibular, and visual balance systems. In this way, the functional abilities of the somatosensory, visual, and vestibular balance systems can be ascertained in comparison to norms established for various ages and heights. CDPP is a useful tool not only in diagnosis and therapy but also in demonstrating to the patient and family the limitations and strengths of the patient under various conditions. We have found CDPP to be particularly useful in setting goals and demonstrating improvement over time. This provides a significant incentive and motivation to the patient that we have not been able to achieve easily in any other way.

Visit Two
Examination of Nonvestibular Systems

The second visit consists mainly of testing the "nonvestibular" body systems (leg strength, cardiovascular, etc.) as well as other factors that could also be contributing to falls. This is best accomplished as a multidisciplinary effort. At the Henry Ford Falls Prevention Clinic, counseling by the team at the end of the visit is considered one of the most effective aspects of the process. Table 5–3 shows a list of the tests as well as who performs these tests. Whoever performs the various tests should be adequately trained and acting within the bounds of their various clinical privileges.

Review of Medical Record (prior to patient visit)

Prior to the second visit, the medical record is reviewed to obtain information on past and ongoing medical issues as well as past and current medications. **Medications** are noted for side effects of dizziness, vertigo, or imbalance. **Ototoxicity** is considered by looking for past issues in which ototoxic agents may have been used such as any infections requiring intravenous antibiotics or cancer treated by chemotherapy. A current list of ototoxic agents may be found in Roland and Rutka (2004). Vestibular test results are reviewed prior to the visit, usually consisting of VNG or ENG and rotational chair report. At this point, prior to the second visit, the Falls Clinic Report is beginning to be compiled so that it can be delivered to the patient and family at the conclusion of the visit.

Table 5–3. Tests Included in Visit Two of the Falls Clinic (with suggested order)

Prior to Visit	Performed By
1. Review of the medical record	Audiologist/Physician
2. Review of vestibular test results	Audiologist
3. Falls Questionnaire (waiting room)	Audiologist
During the Visit (with the patient)	
4. History (General)	Audiologist/Physician
5. Orthostatics	Physician/Audiologist
6. Cognition/Mood assessment	Audiologist/Physician
7. Cerebellar screening	Audiologist/Physician/ Physical therapist
8. Lower extremity strength and feeling	Physical therapist/ Physician/Audiologist
9. Posturography	Audiologist
10. Informal balance and mobility	Audiologist/Physical therapist
11. Neck screening	Physical therapist/ Audiologist/Physician
12. Vision	Audiologist
13. Physical therapy evaluation	Physical therapist
14. Environmental assessment	Physical therapist/Audiologist
15. Risk factor assessment and report	Audiologist (while patient reading safety handout)
16. Counseling session	Audiologist/Physician/ Physical therapist

Previous Medical Conditions

Although falls are usually related to the musculoskeletal, nervous or cardiovascular systems, it is also possible for any system to contribute to or cause falls. For example, falls could even be contributed to by a deficit in the respiratory system if, for example, the condition were severe enough to cause episodic hypoxia with resultant syncope. A review of the systems less likely to contribute to falls can be made by reviewing results of a recent physical examination, obtaining information from the patient, or by performing direct screening. A written history questionnaire, although beneficial, is not considered adequate to accomplish this because falling patients are often poor historians or are unaware of their own status. If results of a recent physical examination are not available, on-site screenings of these less likely systems should be performed.

Generalized Body Weakness

Generalized body weakness, from whatever cause, also predisposes a person to falls. Any health condition that may cause generalized weakness or weakness in the lower extremities should be assessed from chart review and screenings during the falls examination.

Orthostatic Hypotension or Irregular Pulse

Testing for postural hypotension takes several minutes; therefore, it is often neglected in physical examinations unless the patient specifically complains of lightheadedness when standing. Very often we have found that older patients have not communicated this adequately to their doctor and have missed being diagnosed.

Testing is performed by taking the blood pressure after the patient has been lying supine for 5 minutes and again on standing at 1 minute. A drop of 15 to 20 points systolic or an increase in pulse rate of 20 points is significant. Increase in pulse rate is also suggestive of postural hypotension. Although testing while standing after 1 minute is the standard procedure, testing immediately on standing also provides useful information because that is the time frame during which a person will probably fall (immediately after standing). An irregular pulse may also be noted on testing. This is considered clinically significant only if the patient is experiencing lightheadedness. Any irregularities in the pulse are noted.

Cognition and Mood

A screening tests for cognition and mood, which themselves are risk factors for falls, may be conducted conveniently while the patient is lying supine waiting the 5 minutes necessary prior to taking the lying-down blood pressure reading. Cognition may be assessed using portions of or the complete Mini-Mental Status Examination (Folstein, Folstein, & McHugh, 1975) which is a quick, easy assessment of a variety of cognitive functions including short-term memory and language. Mood can be assessed by simply asking whether the patient experiences significant depression. There are also standardized scales available for assessing mood; however, there is evidence that just asking about depression directly is adequate.

Cerebellar Function

Cerebellar dysfunction is a possible cause of imbalance and abnormal gait. The reader is referred to the excellent text by Blumenfeld (2002), especially Chapter 15, for a review of symptoms and tests of cerebellar ataxia. We screen cerebellar function using standard bedside cerebellar tests. These include the finger-nose-finger test, precision finger tap, and heel to shin test. The finger-nose-finger test requires the patient to accurately touch his own nose, then the examiner's outstretched finger, doing so alternately several times. In the precision finger tap test, the patient attempts to tap each finger of a given hand to the thumb tip of the same hand. The heel to shin test requires the patient, while lying supine, to run the heel of one foot down the entire length of the anterior leg of the other side, from knee to ankle.

Lower Extremity Strength and Feeling

Strength

Direct examination should be made of lower extremity **strength**, **feeling**, **morphology**, and **function**. Additional evaluation should be made by chart review and history for other known musculoskeletal disorders that could contribute to falls.

Strength is tested by having the patient apply pressure from the extremity being tested to the examiner's arm or hand. A five-point subjective rating scale (5 being greatest strength) is used by the examiner to assess flexion and extension strength of ankles, knees, and hips. Figures 5–4 and 5–5 show examples of lower extremity strength testing.

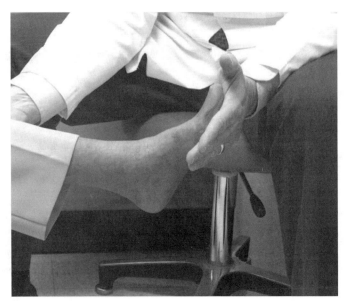

A.

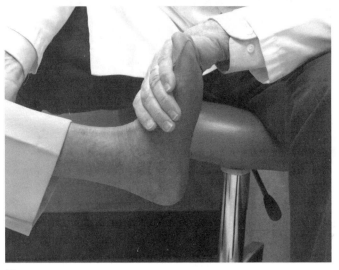

B.

Figure 5–4. Ankle strength testing. While the examiner supports the lower leg, the patient pushes the foot against the examiner's opposing hand (**A**). Strength is evaluated on a subjective 1- to 5-point scale, with 5 being the greatest. Ankle flexion strength is also assessed by having the patient bend the foot upward while the examiner opposes this motion with the hand (**B**).

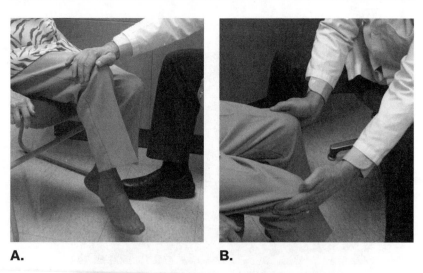

A.   **B.**

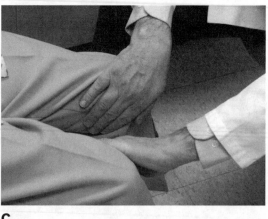

C.

Figure 5–5. Hip strength testing. The patient attempts to keep the foot off the floor while the examiner tries to push the knee down (**A**). In (**B**), the patient attempts to spread the knees against the examiner's hands. In (**C**), the patient attempts to close the knees against the examiner's hands.

Sensation and Proprioception

Neural conduction time is the preferred test of many neurologists for determining peripheral neuropathy. This test is usually performed by a neuroscience laboratory (often the EEG lab) available in many hospitals. Some audiologists alternatively may use somatosensory evoked potentials (SEPs) for this purpose. These tests are only necessary if the patient fails a screening test for neuropathy or if there are complaints of lack of feeling or pain in the legs without previous testing. As this is a common disorder, many patients coming to the Falls Clinic will have already been diagnosed with neuropathy. Neuropathy is especially prevalent in diabetics but may also be common in others. Physical therapists usually perform this type of testing by using light touch applied to areas of the feet and legs, watching for decreased feeling as the stimulus moves lower on the leg, or asymmetry of feeling when comparing right and left.

Screening should be performed using at least two of the following methods:

a. The **"pin prick"** test assesses feeling using a sharp object such as a broken Q-tip applied lightly to the skin of the knee and proceeding downward to the foot. The patient indicates whether the sensation becomes significantly lighter as the stimulus is applied lower and lower on the leg. Also, comparison is made between legs as to the relative intensity of sensation. Except for the area close to the ankle where feeling is typically a bit less, sensation should not be reduced as the pin prick proceeds lower (Figure 5–6).

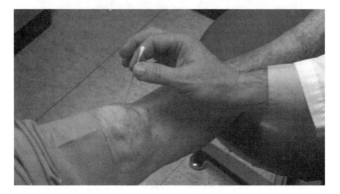

Figure 5–6. Sensation testing (pinprick test). The patient's leg is touched lightly with the broken end of a Q-tip. The patient notes whether there is a generally lessened sensation as the stimulus proceeds down the leg.

b. **Light touch** is an alternative to the pin prick test just covered. Instead of the sharp broken end of a Q-tip, the soft end is used to lightly touch areas of the leg and foot, again comparing upper areas with those going down and comparing left and right.

c. **Tuning fork test.** This test utilizes a low-frequency tuning fork such as 125 Hz applied to the tip of the big toe. Criterion for normal is being able to feel the vibration. The patient should be shown what the vibration feels like by applying the fork first to a more sensitive part of the body such as the wrist. In our experience this test produces many false positives in that persons without significant neuropathy often cannot feel the vibration on the big toe or are unsure (Figure 5-7).

d. **Big toe up or down test.** This test assesses proprioception, which is the ability to determine the spatial location of an appendage, by moving the big toe up or down without the patient looking to determine whether or not the correct position can be determined without looking. The toe should be grasped on the sides rather than top and bottom, otherwise sensation on the skin on the top or bottom of the

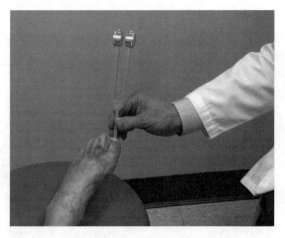

Figure 5-7. Sensation testing (tuning fork test).

toe will give an inadvertent clue to direction. By holding the toe at each side, this clue is equalized more easily. The up or down positions should be randomized in order not to provide further clues to the patient. Abnormalities with muscle function or severe neuropathy could also possibly invalidate proprioception testing.

Morphology

Problems with structure of the feet or legs (morphology) such as deformity, may cause abnormal gait with falls. The feet and legs should be inspected for any gross abnormalities in structure such as missing toes, severe bunion, or other abnormality. Figure 5-8 shows an example of disparate leg length.

Posturography

It is advisable to perform posturography during the second Falls Clinic visit, unless it is needed during the previous vestibular evaluation (VNG/ENG, rotational chair) in order to establish the cause of vertigo. Performing posturography during the second visit is of benefit for demonstrating to the family or patient their particular balance strengths and weaknesses. The scores obtained can also be used for reference at a future follow-up visit as a level to exceed following any rehabilitation measures recommended. This can be a very motivating factor in the patient's progress in improving balance ability assuming that this is possible.

Informal Balance and Mobility Tests (Balance, Gait, and Range of Motion)

In addition to the Romberg, Fukuda, and Gans Sensory Organization Performance Test previously discussed in this chapter, the following methods may be used to assess gait and balance in terms of falls risk. It is wise to use a safety belt or harness on the patient to avoid an accident while testing:

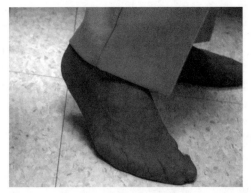

A.

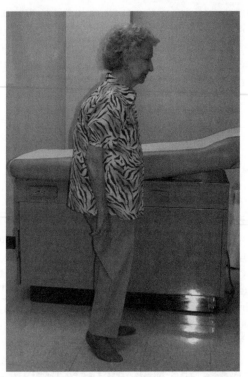

B.

Figure 5–8. Morphology. Example of patient with legs having different length. In this figure (**A** and **B**), while the patient is attempting to stand normally, the right heel remains off the ground.

Tinetti Performance Oriented Mobility Assessment

The Performance Oriented Mobility Assessment (POMA) (Tinetti, 1986), is divided into two parts, balance and gait. Tinetti, in her tests, has proposed a group of criteria that are useful in describing the strengths and weakness of the patient's balance and gait. Rather than using this as a formal test, we observe the patient performing all tasks and describe any abnormal performance in our written evaluation. The Tinetti tasks that we find most useful are shown in Table 5–4. Figure 5–9 shows a patient performing some of the tasks. The main idea is to watch the patient performing everyday tasks such as reaching or turning in place which simulate activities that might lead to falls.

Many of Tinetti's criteria for the assessment of **gait** are also very helpful when describing abnormal gait. Included among the descriptors are, "feet barely clear the floor," "feet pass very close to each other," "gait is not deviating," "arms are not abducted," and so forth. The reader is referred to the original article or easily obtainable summaries for more details. It has been noted recently that the "Tinetti test" has been called by different names and utilized differently by various investigators; therefore, caution should be used when interpreting studies using this test (Kopke & Meyer, 2006).

Table 5–4. "Tinetti" Tasks Used at Henry Ford Falls Clinic

* Reaching up while looking up
* Bending over to pick something up
* Turning a small circle in place in either direction (eyes open)
* Walking straight, turning while walking
* Nudged on the sternum, back, and each shoulder
* Standing up or sitting down in one smooth motion without imbalance
* Looking up while arching the back
* Turning the head far to the side while standing (in either direction)

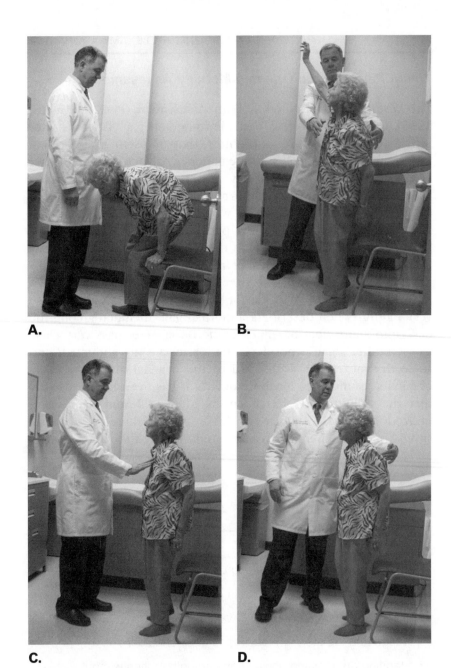

Figure 5–9. Tinetti tasks evaluated as part of the informal balance tests. This figure illustrates examples of the Tinetti tasks, including standing up without imbalance (**A**), reaching up while looking up (**B**), being nudged from the front (**C**), and back (**D**) (nudges should also be done from the side at each shoulder).

"Get Up and Go" Test

In this test (Podsiadlo & Richardson, 1991; Mathias, Nayak, & Isaacs, 1986), the amount of time is determined for a person to rise from sitting, walk 3 meters, return to the chair, and sit down again. The person can use any walking device typically used. Although there is not always agreement among those using the test as to the cut-off time for normal, (10 seconds has been suggested), the greater reason for performing the test is that it gives the examiner an opportunity to observe the patient at his or her worst, that is, when rushing. The fact that the person has to turn at one point in the task is also very telling as there are frequent falls at that point during this test. The examiner should accompany the patient using a safety belt or harness to prevent a potential fall during examination. We have found the Get Up and Go test to be very useful, although not foolproof, in assessing a patient's risk of falls. The test is useful as a way to have the patient rush as quickly as possible, therefore allowing the examiner to see the patient in the situation simulating rushing to answer a doorbell or phone. The examiner watches for instability and unsteadiness while the patient is rushing.

Standing on Foam

Having the patient stand on thick foam with the eyes closed assesses the vestibular system because visual and somatosensory input is eliminated under these conditions leaving only the vestibular sensations intact (Figure 5–10).

Although posturography provides a calibrated mechanism for measuring balance under varying conditions of movable or fixed surface, eyes open or closed, and so forth, assessing the patient's balance while standing on a piece of thick foam has the advantage of more easily demonstrating to the patient his or her own ability to balance under varying visual conditions. Counseling may then be performed at that point. If, for example, the patient with eyes closed falls when standing on the foam, it demonstrates the increased risk on soft surfaces such as thick foam as well as the importance of having adequate lighting such as night lights in darkened rooms.

Dr. Richard Gans, has outlined a standard method of testing the vestibular system function using special high-density foam (obtainable from the American Institute of Balance, Seminole, Florida),

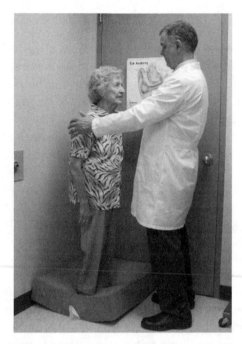

Figure 5–10. Vestibular testing (standing on foam test). The patient attempts to stand on foam (thick enough that the ground cannot be felt) with eyes closed for several seconds. Near falling or falling is considered abnormal; however, at advanced ages, if a person can stand, even if unsteadily, for several seconds with eyes closed, the test is considered negative.

which is called the Gans Sensory Organization Performance Test (SOP). Seven conditions are tested from easiest (standing on the floor with feet together with eyes open) to most difficult (standing on foam with eyes closed).

Neck Screening

The contribution of the neck to balance problems and vertigo has been recognized for many years, but the neck is gaining more and more attention recently. The neck can affect balance in two ways, the nerve pathways to and from the vestibular system, referred to as the cervicovestibular tract, as well as arteries whose blockage causes symptoms of lightheadedness or feeling of impending faint. Such blockage may be due either to internal occlusions such as in carotid artery occlusion or the mechanical pinching off of the blood flow as sometimes occurs in vertebral-basilar artery insufficiency.

Screening for the mechanical blockages can be performed in several ways. Although nystagmus may not be present, symptoms can sometimes be reproduced by having the patient sit upright with the head back and to the side, thereby creating stress on the arteries supplying the head. The position should be obtained for at least 30 seconds, but longer if possible. Instead of asking the patient if he or she is dizzy, ask the patient the more general query, "How do you feel?" Symptoms include headache, nausea, or dizziness that is quite pronounced. If symptoms are only slight, this is probably not significant. Alternative methods shown in some textbooks include placing the patient in the Hallpike position; however, this is more easily confused with benign positional vertigo.

Screening for the neural type of neck vertigo is somewhat challenging. Nystagmus may be produced when the head is turned but if the patient is lying, then this may represent otologic or more central types of nystagmus. Therefore, the presence of nystagmus when the patient is seated is more convincing. VNG/ENG protocols also traditionally differentiate neck disorder from peripheral or central "positional nystagmus" by looking for nystagmus both with the patient lying to the side as well as having the patient only turn the head to the side while lying supine. If the nystagmus is present only with the head to the side but not the whole body, then the neck is implicated. Looking for nystagmus with the patient seated and the head to the side helps to overcome this confusion. As it is possible that this seated position could cause otologic nystagmus just due to the patient's head movement, a preferred method would be to have the patient seated on a movable stool and then, while keeping the head in the same position, turn the body only, thereby creating the same position without having to actually move the head. This method has been proposed by Gans (2006).

Once the neck is implicated on one of these screening tests, it is a much more difficult task to prove this by imaging studies. Such studies are costly and seldom show positive findings. It is this situation that has probably led many otolaryngologists to disbelieve the neck's contribution to vertigo. Many physical therapists take a more practical approach, believing that in many cases muscle tightness leads to pinching of nerves in the neck. Physical therapists cite frequent cases of relieving vertigo by using neck relaxation therapies. Vertebral neck disorders are also implicated in this problem but would not be so amenable to safe or effective physical therapy. In summary, neck problems are likely a common cause of vertigo and balance problems; however, treating them should be done judiciously under close medical supervision after ruling out dangerous spinal disorders that may be dangerous to have therapy performed on.

Vision Testing

Visual acuity of 20/50 (binocular corrected) or poorer itself places an individual at high risk of falls. Visual acuity should be tested with the glasses using both eyes simultaneously. If the person has glasses but never uses them, then test under the condition that is most typical (glasses or no glasses).

    Contrast vision, if abnormal, has also been shown to cause risk of falls due to the inability to see the edges of steps or curbs. The **Melborne Edge Test** (Wolffsohn, Eperjesi, & Napper, 2005) may be used to screen for abnormal contrast vision. A transparent sheet having circles with one half dark in lighter and lighter shades is placed on a light box such as an x-ray viewing box. The patient stands close to the light box and determines the smallest numbered circle for which the dark half can be distinguished. Reading glasses if used by the patient may be used for the test. We use a score of 19 or smaller to indicate normal contrast vision.

Physical Therapy Evaluation and Environmental Assessment

The physical therapy examination assesses balance and gait, strength of ankles, knees, and hips, and sensation of the lower extremities and performs the "Environmental Assessment." The Environmental

Assessment is a list of questions concerning risk factors in the living environment as well as personal habits relating to those.

In our Falls Clinic, the physical therapist arrives near the end of one patient's visit and then sees the next patient at the beginning of the next patient's visit. If there are only two "falls" patients, then the therapist can see them both back to back and then leave. After the physical therapy evaluation, results are related to the audiologist and physician and the three meet to discuss all the findings and recommendations including any recommendations for physical therapy. The physical therapist is often able to obtain information about the patient having fallen that the audiologist or physician were not able to obtain. It is often helpful if the physical therapist can participate in the final counseling portion of the visit but this is not always possible. If not, the physical therapist must give the verbal instructions at the end of the physical therapy portion of the clinic visit. The physical therapist's presence during the final counseling portion of the examination lends credence to the recommendations that are given. This group model is often beneficial as explained later in this chapter.

Counseling Session

The final counseling session occurs at the end of the Falls Clinic visit, ideally with the team and family members attending. In this final portion of the visit, final results are conveyed along with a hard copy of the report if possible. The aim of such a report is to suggest possible solutions for each of the three major causes of falls, medical, behavioral, and extrinsic. It is usually possible to complete this report during the team consultation just prior to the counseling session. If it is not possible to finish the report at the visit, the report can be mailed later. At the least, a written list of immediate recommendations should be given the patient or family member on leaving the visit so that immediate changes such as use of a walker or other safety features may be implemented as soon as possible.

The final counseling session is perhaps the most useful aspect of the Falls Clinic. It is gratifying to watch the decisions being made by the patient and family in this group session of the visit. It is not uncommon to decide on changes in living arrangements or modifications of the physical surroundings of the patient. Often, the accompanying family member will realize for the first time that their loved one is falling frequently. When all of the patient's problems have been listed and the needed modifications of the home outlined, family members may realize that their loved one is unlikely to comply with the suggestions. This further motivates a more substantial change in living arrangements, which often occurs in these sessions.

Recommendation for the use of a walker or other assistive device is also made during this portion of the visit. As can be imagined, this recommendation is not usually met with approval by the patient. But reminding the patient that such a measure will often prolong independence and being confronted by the group often convinces the patient of the wisdom in using a walker.

The Falls Clinic allows for direct observation of the patient walking and doing things that simulate falling situations. For example, the Tinetti criteria for gait and balance have the patient reach high arching the back, turning a tight circle in place, picking up something from the ground, and other actions which may precipitate a fall. The patient wears a safety harness, which the tester can hold onto during these assessments. Very often, by observing the patient in these circumstances, the cause of falls becomes obvious. For example, consider a patient whose legs are found to be very weak and whose reaction times for the feet are very slow. The complaint is that the patient falls whenever bending forward. Although it would be logical to think of possible orthostatic changes in blood pressure while bending, or benign positional vertigo causing an imbalance while bending over, if tests for these are negative, then it appears obvious by observing the patient that falling forward is a simple matter of the feet and legs not having the strength or quickness to arrest the forward motion, thus the patient falls forward. This demonstrates the value of a comprehensive evaluation by a single team of clinicians so that all the information obtained can be integrated in order to arrive at the proper conclusion.

As mentioned above, having the assessment team as a group present in the counseling session is an impressive way to demonstrate consensus of the findings and stresses the importance of following recommendations for the safety of the patient. On occasion, the assistance of a social worker is sought by the clinician when elder abuse, neglect, or inability to care for oneself is obvious. Such cases, in which it becomes apparent that a patient is being taken advantage of financially by a nonrelative, has no close relative or agency to look in on them, or is mentally incompetent of self-care should be referred to a social worker or other agency as the law may dictate.

It is our philosophy to stress the positive and offer hope and solutions whenever possible. When testing older individuals, quite a long list of abnormal results often emerges, some of which may not have much to do with the patient's falling. The goal is to provide a list of a few prioritized problems, "falls risk factors," that can be addressed by the patient with some success. In some cases, however, it becomes apparent that the patient is likely to fall again, as he or she has fallen several times in the past and perhaps is not willing to comply with the recommendations. In that case, it is sometimes best to focus more on injury prevention rather than the unlikely goal of eliminating all falls. Protective clothing, hip protectors, or other injury preventive devices may be the best solution in such cases. Every individual presents with a slightly different set of circumstances and should be dealt with in a customized manner.

Rationale for the Falls Clinic

An individual "falls examination" has been shown by several studies to be an important component of falls prevention. In their "Guidelines for the Prevention of Falls in Older Persons" published in 2001, the Joint Panel on Falls Prevention consisting of members from the American Geriatrics Society, British Geriatrics Society, and American Academy of Orthopaedic Surgeons states that a "fall-related assessment" coupled with intervention is likely to reduce the probability of falls. Individual medical evaluation is necessary because the causes of falls are so varied, originating from a broad range of disorders.

Determining the cause of falls is a challenging endeavor requiring more than a cursory examination. With many fallers being older individuals having several medical problems that could be causing their falls, such patients are sometimes labeled simply as having "multifactorial" causes of falls. Leaving it at that is a lackadaisical approach because it implies that the patient has a variety of medical problems with no way of knowing the main cause of the falls. Such labeling also ascribes a kind of hopelessness to the situation. In our experience, however, taking the necessary time needed to perform tests often will reveal a **main cause** of the falls or at least result in a **prioritized list** of causes. If this can be accomplished, finding ways of preventing falls is much easier. Because the causes of falls cover several areas of expertise, we employ a **team approach** when possible. Our outpatient-based Falls Prevention Clinic allows the audiologist to work in conjunction with an otolaryngologist or other referring physician prior to the Falls Clinic visit and an internal medicine specialist and physical therapist during the visit. Results of the prior balance function test, consisting of the vestibular tests VNG/ENG and rotational chair, are available at the visit.

The goal of the falls examination is to obtain information in the three areas: medical causes, circumstances surrounding falls and "fall risk factors." To accomplish this, the falls examination obtains information in the following categories:

1. **Systems assessment** consisting of a medical evaluation of the body systems most likely to cause falls: **cardiovascular, musculoskeletal, and nervous systems,** as well as any **other ongoing medical problems** potentially contributing to falls. Such a "physiologic" approach to falls prediction has been pioneered by Lord and colleagues and is described in a recent paper, which influenced our clinic's work (Lord, Menz, & Tiedemann, 2003).

2. **Falls descriptions** consisting of interviewing the patient to explore the circumstances surrounding specific falls. The patient as well as any eyewitnesses to falls should be thoroughly interviewed so that the causes of falls, whether behavioral, physiologic, or environmental, may be ascertained.

3. **Assessment of falls risk factors** consisting of an assessment of **environmental** and **behavioral** "risk factors" that are known to cause increased risk of falls such as the patient having to climb stairs to the sleeping quarters.

Information for the above three categories does not have to be obtained in the order listed or all at once. For example, specific questions regarding falls descriptions and risk factors (items 2 and 3 above) may be asked during the physical portions of the examination when the patient is attempting to perform certain tasks such as walking or reaching up. The history is most effectively obtained during both the beginning portion and ending portion of the examination. A general history before the examination is necessary for the tester to know what to look for. Specific information is easier to obtain during the examination itself, particularly regarding circumstances of falls, because the tester has seen the patient's capabilities and knows how to better frame certain questions and incorporate this information later into the recommendations.

Testing Order

Tests of the Falls Clinic visit may be efficiently performed in the order shown on the forms in Appendix B (see the templates of forms for rough data and the final report in Appendix B). Details regarding the individual tests are provided in the following section. The order shown is, of course, not mandatory but provides several worthwhile features. Time is saved by reviewing the chart and possible medical effects on dizziness prior to the visit. It is the goal to give the patient a hard copy of the report on leaving the evaluation. This provides several advantages. Giving the patient a hard copy allows the patient to immediately put into practice the suggestions and recommendations received. By providing the patient with a copy, there is no misunderstanding the instructions or recommendations. These instructions and recommendations may be extensive and too hard to remember unless a written copy is provided. If there is no time to provide the entire report, at least a list of recommendations should be provided as the patient leaves. Also, giving the patient a hard copy of the report may eliminate the need for other copies to be sent to other health care providers. Patients who are experiencing falls are often seeing several other health care providers and the hard copy can eliminate a lot of work for the clinician.

The cognitive examination and mood examination may be performed while the patient is lying supine during the 5-minute waiting period before performing the orthostatic blood pressure testing.

At the end of the examination, a counseling session is given with as many of the clinicians present as possible. Results and recommendations are presented to the patient and family. Decisions made in these sessions include change of living arrangements, use of a walker or cane, or recommendation for physical therapy either as an outpatient or in the home.

Triage of the Dizzy Patient

Recognizing that a multitude of disorders can cause "dizziness," the goals of triage need to be stated. For purposes of many otolaryngology or audiology clinics, the goal is to find all "vestibular" patients and eliminate all others who can be treated by the more appropriate specialty. Audiologist's closest allies in purpose, otolaryngologists, have the additional motivation for wanting to identify "true vestibular" cases, namely, they are inundated with dizzy patients who are not appropriately treated by their specialty. Many patients, whose primary causes of dizziness are blood pressure or medication issues, are mistakenly diverted to ENT as the clinic of choice as though the otolaryngologist desires to see any type of dizzy patient.

The elements of a minimal triage program to screen for vestibular etiology include the screening protocol already described early in this chapter, plus testing for orthostatic hypotension.

Personnel

The personnel involved may consist of those from a variety of specialties, but there should be expertise in the areas described below. Example specialists are provided for each area of expertise; however, other professionals could possibly provide these assessments if properly trained and there are no prohibitive "scope of practice" or licensing issues. The suggested personnel listed in Table 5-3 are modifiable and there is room for variations in personnel chosen to perform the various assessments provided they are qualified.

Personnel for "General Medical" Assessment

One of the potential strengths of a multidisciplinary falls clinic is that there is contribution by more than one physician specialty. An internal medicine specialist is a good choice for the falls clinic because the problems commonly encountered in falling individuals often include issues of blood pressure, cardiology, or medication. Internal medicine physicians are well prepared in these areas as well as in areas of general medical disorders affecting strength and feeling in the lower extremities such as diabetes. Neurologists, and in some cases family practice specialists, are also a good choice. Having an otolaryngologist perform all of these assessments is often impractical due to either a lack of interest or up-to-date experience in these areas. Some otolaryngologists, however, enjoy the general medical and vestibular aspects of dizziness and some non-surgical otolaryngologists seek such patients. In a large training hospital or clinic, it is sometimes possible to elicit the help of medical residents in internal medicine or neurology. Another option is to utilize physician assistants or nurse practitioners who are trained in these areas.

The duties of the specialist performing the "general medical" assessment include review of the prior and current ongoing medical issues as they may relate to falls and review of appropriateness of all medications as they either may affect balance directly as a side effect, or indirectly as body functions are affected by them.

In the Henry Ford Hospital Falls Prevention Clinic, the internal medicine specialist is a very valuable component of the "falls clinic" team. Very often it is discovered that the patient is on too many or too high dosage of blood pressure medications, that there is an abnormal heart rate or rhythm, or that some aspect of the patient's health has been overlooked. These oversights probably occur when the patient takes charge of his or her own medical management instead of having a single "primary physician" manage the patient. Patients sometimes hop from one health system to another in search of a solution. In other instances, the patient's own doctors overlook general health issues because the patient may have a specific challenging disorder that is demanding all of the attention. At our clinic, this physician is one of the internal medicine residents who are currently completing a geriatric medicine rotation. In some clinics, a more permanent physician serves as "Medical Director." In many settings, this arrangement may also satisfy insurance requirements. The physician is an invaluable member of the team due to the varied medical causes causing or contributing to falls. The internal medicine specialty works well because fallers often have blood pressure, cardiovascular, or general medical issues that are easily solved by doctors within this specialty. Other specialties could also fulfill this role. The importance of testing for blood pressure, neuropathy, and strength at the Falls Clinic visit is evidenced by the fact that the physician is often surprised at the number of times issues such as orthostasis and neuropathy have been previously missed on these patients. This may be because these problems were not expressed to the patient's doctor as a primary complaint. Also, testing for these issues adds considerable time to a physical examination.

If the patient fails the neuropathy screening and is previously not diagnosed with this disorder, the patient is sent for neural conduction time testing, usually the same day.

Personnel for Vestibular and Oculomotor Assessment

Traditionally, audiologists and vestibular physiologists are those having the greatest role in vestibular testing by virtue of their extensive training and experience. However, not all audiologists are given in-depth training specifically in vestibular testing, although most have had extensive coursework in the area. Audiologists without lengthy experience or training can receive on-site vestibular coursework fairly easily through several vestibular training clinics and workshops. In some cases, those in other fields have also had extensive training, such as physical therapists or physicians who have become interested specifically in balance and vestibular testing. Although not as frequently well trained in vestibular testing, physical therapists receive the greatest training and experience in general balance assessment as well as rehabilitation. During the past few years, this picture has begun to change. There is overlap in expertise for physical therapists, audiologists, and physicians in the areas of vestibular and balance as well as in rehabilitation. In some cases, there is competition for patients in these areas. In other settings, however, there is increased collaboration among these specialists. For example, at Henry Ford Hospital Falls Prevention Clinic, the audiologist serves as clinic coordinator, performing vestibular testing and combining data from the other tests. The internal medicine physician performs the "general medicine" assessment, and the physical therapist performs the lower extremity and gait assessments as well as recommends physical therapy when appropriate.

Physical Therapist

The physical therapist arrives toward the end of the visit and receives a briefing by the audiologist regarding the findings of the examination so far. After the physical therapist's examination which covers issues of home safety, balance, gait, strength, and sensation issues, these results are conveyed to the audiologist. At this point, a brief conference is held by the team, the report is finalized, and then the team meets with the patient. Usually, the final report is presented at this time and further recommendations are made.

Because falls are caused by a variety of disorders, a multidisciplinary falls clinic has the greatest potential for properly diagnosing and treating the underlying medical causes of falls. It is our philosophy that as falls can be caused by a variety of body systems, the most efficient and effective type of falls clinic would be multidisciplinary.

Advantages of Establishing a "Falls Clinic"

The popularity of "falls clinics" is rapidly growing. Due to the increasing number of patients who fall and potential dire consequences of falls, such clinics are viewed as a potential solution to the problem (see Chapter 1). Multidisciplinary falls clinics are advantageous to the patient because there can be one central clinic addressing falls, without which the patient must make numerous doctor visits in order to discover the cause of the falls. Falls clinics also have the potential to become extremely popular among referring doctors for several reasons. One type of faller, the "dizzy patient," is looked on by many physicians as less desirable to the practice because of the extra time needed for assessment. Also, because falls are caused by a multiplicity of disorders sharing the same vague symptoms, there are often a high percentage of cases in which the disorder is found to be outside the physician's area of specialization. Because falls clinics usually incorporate a rehabilitation component, falls clinics are viewed by many physicians and potential patients as a means of providing both an assessment of the problem as well as a solution. Prior to the newer rehabilitation strategies now available, unless there was a specific acute disorder, there was not much that could be done to help the patient, leaving both the physician and patient frustrated. Multispecialty falls clinics have been shown to be effective in identifying causes and reducing falls by a recent study of the Henry Ford Falls Prevention Clinic. Establishing a falls clinic, however, is somewhat complex and, therefore, requires adequate planning for success.

Practice Benefits of a "Falls Clinic"

Beyond the obvious benefits to the falling patient, there are many benefits to the overall success of the audiology practice of providing a "falls clinic." The problem of falls is so pervasive in our society that the concept of a falls clinic draws immediate attention and opens up various opportunities from a publicity and marketing standpoint. In the Henry Ford Health System, the announcement of the Falls Prevention Clinic drew immediate attention from the marketing department who publicized the clinic in newsletters and offers to give talks. In our highly competitive health care market, hospitals and other institutions are constantly looking for ways to improve their image and demonstrate the services they provide their customers. The message of preventive medicine provides a positive caring image. These and other opportunities provide ways for increased interaction between audiologists and other professionals thereby providing a means of educating others on what we do. The name "falls clinic" presents a very practical image to the concept of balance testing. This name conveys the message of the outcome hoped for and states that problem is being solved rather than just offering tests of balance.

An audiology-based Falls Clinic is successful because it is well positioned to determine why a patient is falling and provides solutions to such falls through measures such as vestibular rehabilitation. But why is an *audiology-based* clinic particularly suited to these ends? First, most patients fall because they are either dizzy or have a balance problem, with a smaller percentage of fallers having other primary causes of their falls such as movement disorders, generalized weakness, or cardiogenic problems. Audiologists often are specifically trained to assess balance and dizziness symptoms. But are they suited to treat such dizziness and balance issues? The majority of cases of dizziness or associated balance abnormalities are caused by benign paroxysmal positional vertigo (BPPV), uncompensated vestibulopathy of nonspecific origin, or bilateral vestibular weakness, with only a small percentage of cases being attributed to "medically treatable" causes such as Ménière's disease. Audiologists not only have expertise in the treatment of BPPV and uncompensated vestibulopathy, but such treatment is within their scope of practice according to many accrediting organizations and licensing bodies. Very recently, audiologists now report a high degree of success both for discovering the cause of dizziness and treating it. This recent success is due to two major new factors: (1) the testing of patients with higher speed head rotation measures than previously obtainable, and (2) the success of recent vestibular rehabilitation methods that audiologists can employ.

Summary

Successful multispecialty falls clinics will have the following elements: well-trained personnel having expertise from various specialties, equipment capable of assessing the balance system, adequate facilities, and adequate sources of referrals.

Falls prevention clinics utilize the philosophy that a team approach that addresses all potentially contributing body systems is the most efficient and effective approach to the medical intervention of falls prevention. This falls clinic can be a valuable addition to the services offered by our health system and has been shown by recent studies to be effective in reducing the number of falls in most patients attending.

References

Blumenfeld, H. (2002). *Neuroanatomy through clinical cases* (chap 15). Sunderland, MA: Sinauer Associates.

El-Kashlan, H. K., Shepard, N. T., Asher, A. M., Smith-Wheelock, M., & Telian, S. A. (1998). Evaluation of clinical measures of equilibrium. *Laryngoscope, 108*(3), 311–319.

Folstein, M. F., Folstein, S. E., & McHugh, P. R. (1975). Mini-Mental State: A practical method for grading the state of patients for the clinician. *Journal of Psychiatric Research, 12*, 189–198.

Fukuda, T. (1959). The stepping test: Two phases of the labyrinthine reflex. *Acta Otolaryngologica, 50*(2), 95–108.

Fukuda, T. (1984). *Statokinetic reflexes in equilibrium and movement.* Tokyo: University of Tokyo Press.

Fukushima, H., & Hinoki, M. (1985). Role of cervical and lumbar proprioceptors during stepping: an electromyographic study of the muscular activities of the lower limbs. *Acta Otolaryngologica (Stockh)*, Suppl. 419, 91-105.

Gans, R. (2006). *Vestibular rehabilitation: Protocols and programs* (rev. ed.). Seminole, FL: American Institute of Balance.

Gordon, C. R., Fletcher, W. A., Jones, G. M., & Block, E. W. (1995a). Is the stepping test a specific indicator of vestibulospinal function? *Neurology, 45*, 2035-2037.

Gordon, C. R., Fletcher, W. A., Jones, GM, & Block, E. W. (1995b). Adaptive plasticity in the control of locomotor trajectory. *Experimental Brain Research, 102*, 540-545.

Hain, T. C., Fetter, M., & Zee, D,S. (1987). Head-shaking nystagmus in unilateral peripheral vestibular lesions. *American Journal of Otolaryngology, 8*, 36-47.

Halmagyi, G. M., & Curthoys, I. S. (1998). A clinical sign of canal paresis. *Archives of Neurology, 45*(7), 737-739.

Herdman, S. (2004, February). Optimizing the sensitivity of the head thrust test for identifying vestibular hypofunction. Research report. *Physical Therapy, 84*(2), 151-158.

Khasnis, A., & Gokula, R. (2003). Romberg's test. *Journal of Postgraduate Medicine, 49*(2), 169-172.

Kopke, S., & Meyer, G. (2006). The Tinetti test: Babylon in geriatric assessment. *Archives of Gerontology and Geriatrics, 39*(4), 288-291.

Lord, S. R., Menz, H. B., & Tiedemann, A. (2003). A physiological profile approach to falls risk assessment and prevention. *Physical Therapy, 83*(3), 237-252.

Mathias, S., Nayak, U., & Isaacs B. (1986). Balance in elderly patients: The "Get-up and Go" test. *Archives of Physical and Medical Rehabilitation, 67*, 387-389.

Minor, L. B., Cremer, P. D., Carey, J. P., et al. (2001). Symptoms and signs in superior canal dehiscence syndrome. *Annals of the New York Academy of Sciences, 942*, 259-273.

Podsiadlo, D., & Richardson, S. (1991). The timed "Up and Go": A test of basic functional mobility for frail elderly persons. *Journal of the American Geriatric Society, 39*, 142-148.

Roland, P. S., & Rutka, J. A. (2004). *Ototoxicity.* London: BC Decker.

Tinetti, M. E. (1986). Performance-oriented assessment of mobility problems in elderly patients. *Journal of the American Geriatrics Society, 34*, 119-126.

Toper, A. K., Maki, B. E., & Holliday, P. J.(1993). Are activity-based assessments of balance and gait in the elderly predictive of risk of falling and/or type of fall? *Journal of the American Geriatric Society*, *41*, 479–487.

Viirre, E,, Purcell, I., & Baloh, R. W. (2005). The Dix-Hallpike test and the canalith repositioning maneuver. *Laryngoscope*, *115*(1), 184–187.

Wei, D., Hain, T. C., & Proctor, L. (1989). Head-shaking nystagmus: associations with canal paresis and hearing loss. *Acta Otologologica*, *108*, 362–367.

Wolffsohn, J. S., Eperjesi, F., & Napper, G. (2005). Evaluation of Melbourne Edge Test contrast sensitivity measures in the visually impaired. *Ophthalmic and Physiological Optics*, *25*(4), 371–374.

Wrisley. D. M., & Whitney, S. L. (2004). The effect of foot position on the modified clinical test of sensory interaction. *Archives of Physical Medicine and Rehabilitation*, *85*(2), 335–338.

CHAPTER 6

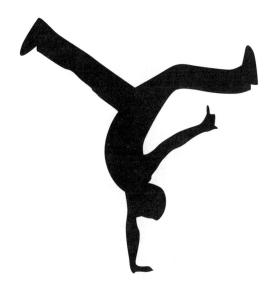

Preventing Falls

The main premise of this book is that falling can be prevented in most patients. The reader is referred to Chapter 7, where specific falls prevention strategies are discussed for hospital and nursing home patients.

Our experience with hundreds of falling patients has taught us that preventing falls is more a behavioral issue than a medical one. This is a bold statement and therefore deserves explanation. Although certain medical conditions can be corrected, in many older individuals this is not always possible; therefore, modifying the patient's behaviors or environment is usually the most effective falls prevention measure. This chapter divides the topic of falls prevention into its three major components, medical intervention, modifying behavior, and education. Also included are the important topics of **environmental modification**, **home safety**, and **walking equipment**. To begin, we discuss what is usually the most important falls prevention measure, modifying the behavior of the patient.

Modifying Behavior

Martha

Martha's case helps to illustrate the importance of behavioral considerations in reducing falls risk. Martha, a healthy looking 85-year-old, lives with her husband in the home they have occupied for years. Unfortunately, Martha has been experiencing an increasing number of falls in the past year, found to be due to a vestibular deficit of unknown etiology. She states that she "walks like a drunk," and observing the patient, she does indeed have a staggering gait especially when turning, starting, or stopping. The vestibular deficit may have been due to an ototoxic medication that permanently reduced the function of both inner ear balance organs. Rehabilitation with a physical therapist for gait and balance training has not improved her gait very much, nor has more specific "vestibular rehabilitation" carried out over a period of several months. Martha is strong for her age, is not overweight, and has no specific medical problems adding to her imbalance other than a mild drop in blood pressure when first standing. This has been improved through adjustments of her blood pressure medications. There are no other significant medical risk factors for falls.

During the second visit to the Falls Clinic, where more practical assessment is made of balance, gait, stair climbing, and mobility functions (see Chapter 5 for description of the tests employed during the Falls Clinic Visit 2), it was noted that the patient's performance on most bedside balance tests was fairly normal, the exception being standing on foam with eyes closed, which she could not do, and the gait assessment already described during which she would easily stagger. Her general appearance while walking was of a person on the brink of falling at any moment. During the observation of the patient's gait, a longer than usual period of observation was taken with the patient. This allowed the opportunity to observe the patient while walking during small distractions, turning corners, becoming somewhat fatigued, stopping, and turning to go back to the examination room. The most significant observation made was that the patient had the habit of walking quickly, turning quickly, and generally rushing.

She stated that walking was easier when she walked faster than when walking slower. This is often noted by patients having abnormal balance, being similar to the experience of riding a bicycle very slowly, which can make that task more difficult. Further discussion with the patient and her daughter revealed that her habit of rushing was more of a general personality trait than just a new recent behavior. Even more disturbing was the revelation that she carries clothing down the stairs to the basement where her washer is, and often is unable to see the steps while walking, which causes her to have to count the steps when going down. She admitted to having thought she was at the bottom when she still had a step to go. Both the patient and her daughter refused to consider moving the washer to the main level, stating the reasons that there would not be room as well as the lack of proper plumbing. The patient also operates her car alone, does not carry a cell phone, and is not considering moving into a more age-appropriate and safe dwelling. There was a discussion of the advantages of considering moving but it was doubtful that this would occur in the near future, despite our observation that sometimes it is easier to move before a crisis occurs. Her main objection was that her husband would be unwilling to move because he has so many personal belongings such as tools and other items that he has been collecting over the years. She also admits to having a large amount of personal items. With the goal being a safer environment, not necessarily a smaller one, we asked if they had considered moving to a larger but single story home. This suggestion did seem to make an impression on the patient. In our experience, simply moving into "assisted living" is not always the best or only solution. A better goal, if available, is to have the person live as independently as possible; however, this does require safety modifications to the home, which often includes rearranging the contents of the home for safety. This may include placing objects lower in cabinets, installing grab bars and extra lighting, as well as other features. Although this is a tedious task, the benefits in the long run may be added extra years of independence and freedom from injury.

Martha's case demonstrates an example of a person whose falling can be largely **controlled by changing her daily habits** and living arrangements. Unfortunately, Martha lacked the flexibility to even consider such changes. Despite our counseling and providing lists of safety features to improve the home, Martha is on the path to almost certain continued falls and possible injury. In contrast, we have seen many patients in similar situations who have been willing to make major home modifications or even change living locations to prevent falls and otherwise improve their living situation.

Although unwilling to make a major move, if she had been more willing to change her current environments, the most effective measures would have included moving the washer to the main level, rearranging items on top or bottom shelves to be at a level that would not require her to reach high or low, and making other home modifications for safety such as adding grab bars in appropriate places and having her carry a cell phone when driving. Discussions of such topics among the family often begin during the counseling portion of the Falls Clinic visit.

Changing Contents of the Home Changes Behavior

A motto in interior design is "form follows function." A motto in falls prevention could be somewhat the opposite, "function follows form," or translated more clearly, "safe behavior follows environmental change." Although changing behaviors is a worthy goal, and easier said than done, the good news is that simply changing the contents of the home often results in the desired behavior changes. For example, changing Martha's lifelong behavior of rushing would have been difficult; however, moving the washer to the main floor would eliminate her risky behavior of carrying clothes up and down the stairs. Similarly, moving small items to lower shelves and placing additional furniture in open areas that can be held onto or fallen against eliminates the behaviors of reaching high and avoids the behavior of walking unassisted in large open areas. Most importantly, removing unsafe items such as low-lying furniture, which can be fallen onto and broken, eliminates an unsafe situation. Furniture, which should be plentiful in a faller's home, should be waist high or higher.

The Need to Change Living Locations

Despite the efforts for independence, at a certain point for a patient with deteriorating health, it may be necessary to consider a change in living location. This often improves the patient's condition generally and decreases the number of falls because the person is being helped with risky behaviors and greater attention can be given to home safety features.

Family members often discuss these changes in living arrangements well before the change is made. Conversations often begin before health crises occur, with discussions centering on what the patient's future expectations are regarding "retirement communities," assisted living, or nursing homes. From a falls prevention standpoint, living alone, or even as an aging couple, at some point becomes an increasingly risky endeavor. The range of activities required for living completely independently involves cleaning, cooking, carrying groceries, and rearranging household items, all of which require a great deal of movement, bending, and reaching. These activities hold a certain amount of risk. On the other hand, these activities do involve beneficial exercise as well as psychological benefits, which help an individual stay healthy. Therefore, it should be the goal to keep people independent as long as it is reasonably safe to do so, but to make the environment a safe one. The next section discusses moving issues, the aim being to make families aware of the important issues involved in these difficult decisions.

The Closer the Better

If a person is at high risk for falls, short of moving in with a relative or friend, the next best thing is to live as close as possible to some concerned party. The simple reason for this is that activities that are difficult or risky can be assisted by others who are close at hand. If the closest relative or friend lives in a different city, there is little likelihood of the at risk person asking for help or obtaining it. If, in contrast, someone responsible is right next door, there is a much higher likelihood of the help occurring. Nonetheless, living alone is still far more dangerous than living with a responsible person. At some point, most people will simply need to have close supervision for at least part of the day. It should be remembered that our discussion concerns mainly the issue of falling; however, the issues of falling often go hand in hand with other significant health problems. Therefore, these principles may also apply to those with other general health issues.

When Is It Time to Move?

When considering falling as a criterion for the need to move, a key question must be answered: Does the falling represent a condition that is likely to continue and become worse, or is the falling due to a medical condition that is likely to pass or be treatable? This is where a visit to the "Falls Clinic" as described in this book is useful. In some cases, falling is caused by a transitory or curable condition such as inner ear (vestibular) disorder; however, when such an ailment occurs late in life, it may be interpreted as simply part of getting old and, therefore, that nothing can be done. In other cases, however, falls do represent the gradual deterioration in which one or more worsening health issues are contributing to an increasing number of falls. A multidisciplinary falls clinic can help to distinguish between these two situations and offer therapy or other treatment as well as aid in the decisions regarding moving.

It is likely time to consider a move when falls are frequent or causing injury. In our experience interviewing fallers, a person usually falls many times before telling anyone this is happening. If an older person mentions that he or she "fell the other day," this usually means that there have been several falls. Once the home has been modified with grab bars and the other safety features mentioned in this book, beyond this, there is little that will occur in the patient's own home to reduce the number of falls. Considering a move is a logical next step.

The attitude of aging individuals about moving changes over time. In their late fifties or early sixties, there may be a feeling of strong independence. However, in a person's seventies, thoughts of being closer to family, "just in case I need them," start to develop. In a person's eighties, there is typically an acute awareness of frailties. Sometimes a self-deception is present at this point where the person may think, "I need some help occasionally" when the reality is that true independent living is seldom actually occurring. It is human nature to think of ourselves as being more independent than we really are. Often, an older individual will be living with family members, doing little of their own cooking, cleaning, or washing, and still consider themselves as performing most of their own maintenance. Admittedly, the decision to move in with a relative is often not difficult for the aging person, but it may be more difficult for the family or person who would become the caretaker.

Where to Move?

Several options present themselves for the family considering helping their relative move to a safer location. "Assisted living" often is considered. This option is defined as a facility in which constant supervision is close at hand, and meals or other common needs such as help with bathing are attended to. However, persons with any major medical problem are often excluded by either the facility's regulations or by law in the state of residence. At a certain point in the seriousness of the condition, persons will be excluded from eligibility in assisted living. More importantly, families are often disappointed to find that just as much time is spent attending to the needs of their relative in assisted living. Frequently, daily visits are required to take care of all the medical, business, or personal needs of the patient. In this regard, having the person closer at hand is an advantage. Also, not everyone adjusts to assisted living. Those who are socially oriented and enjoy making new friendships do well in such an environment. Many people, however, as they grow older enjoy their privacy to an increasing degree and become less social than previously. In these cases, the personality of the patient should be considered. Some patients will feign acceptance of the living situation in order not to be a burden on the family. Assessing the patient's personality and past habits will help determine the potential success of assisted living. Because assisted living facilities and nursing homes are in the business of making money, simply relying on the opinion of the facility's administrators or even the nursing staff regarding the success of the transition is not a reliable way of assessing how the situation is going. There is a strong desire by the facility to make the situation appear successful. Timing is also a consideration, as what may be unacceptable at one time of life, may be thought of as perfectly acceptable at another time. Also, the order of progression from one level of care to another may not always be typical in that some persons will go from their own homes to assisted living to skilled nursing facilities, whereas others may bounce back with better health and then go back to a less supervised environment, even their own homes again. The family may be the only ones who realize the changing condition of the patient in terms of being able to once again leave assisted living and go back to a greater level of independence. This is sometimes the case with hip fractures, which were once considered the "beginning of the end," but now are rehabilitated commonly in persons easily into their nineties. Despite this seeming hodgepodge of choices and situations, there is still room for planning the course of future events, especially if such planning is begun early.

Early Planning

We compare two people who represent opposite ends of the spectrum in terms of living safely and independently as it relates to their differing personalities and lifestyles.

Ardelle, Age 90

Ardelle, a 90-year-old female, lives with her son and daughter-in-law. She keeps to herself in her own three rooms within their home, joining her son and daughter-in-law mainly for meals or at odd times during the day. Ardelle is perfectly happy with her own privacy, is not much of a mixer socially, but mainly enjoys her own close family members. How did she arrive at this successful living situation? Previous planning had at least something to do with the situation. In her mid-seventies, Ardelle had been living with her similarly healthy husband, John, in a separate city away from other family members. Their son and his wife lived in a city approximately 45 miles away, a distance slightly too far to permit daily visits by the family. Discussions began between John and Ardelle and her children concerning the advantages of moving to the city where the children were. A move at this relatively young age would allow them to still live in their own house and, more significantly, stay in it longer because there would be closer help. Such a decision, **to make a major move at a fairly young age, would pro-**

vide a greater chance for successful adjustment to a new home and therefore allow independence for a longer period of time. The plan worked in that for a number of years, the move did allow for the expected advantages in terms of longer independence. In time, however, John became ill with heart disease and gradually deteriorated over a period of several years. Ardelle, meanwhile, now 83 began to lose weight and seemed strained taking care of her husband. Still, the couple got by mainly because the son and daughter-in-law, who now lived within a few blocks, were able to help in terms of meals being brought in as well as helping to perform other necessary tasks.

Ardelle did, however, continue to lose more weight and ultimately fell, breaking a hip. Although she considered this a sign of her impending demise, the rehabilitation went better than she expected and she was able to leave the rehabilitation facility rather quickly. Without Ardelle, however, John was moved to an assisted-living facility. Ardelle joined her husband there but within a couple of weeks it was apparent that things were not going well. Ardelle especially was unhappy living there, being used to her more comfortable home and the greater privacy it offered. John and Ardelle were determined to return to their own home, and with Ardelle's improving condition, this seemed feasible. After returning home, the son and daughter-in-law were now less pleased with the situation than they were during the assisted-living period. The couple really needed more help than they could reasonably offer. Their needs included helping John with bathing and dressing as well as cooking. These daily duties were beyond what could be offered by their children. A live-in nurse's aid was sought. The "nurse" that was finally obtained ended up costing about the same as assisted living, but Ardelle felt that the benefits of being in their own home made it worthwhile. In about one year, John unfortunately passed away, having spent a few weeks in a nursing home, and finally, a few days at home under the care of a hospice nurse. Ardelle, now alone, managed to adjust and even gained some weight being under less stress taking care of her ailing husband. After several more months, however, Ardelle began to experience a few falls. The children were now beginning to realize that she was not really eating as well as she stated. Then, when the son was transferred by his job to another state, it was decided to take Ardelle along. She is now living more successfully and happily with her son and daughter-in-law.

Irene, Age 86

Irene, a widow of 12 years, lives in her own condo. It is a single level duplex-style home with a tiny yard that is maintained by the management who also take care of snow removal and maintenance of the outer aspects of the building. Irene is responsible only for maintaining the inside of the home. This particular condominium facility is home to several others of her age group but is not exclusively a "retirement community"; in fact, the person sharing her building in the adjoining condo is a young single man. Irene is unusually active physically, having enjoyed sports over her lifetime including golf and bowling. She is a "mixer" socially and would prefer being with people on a daily basis than being alone. Her recent activities and hobbies include golf weekly on a "3 par" course and bowling weekly in a senior league. Irene still drives, which allows her more easily to also belong to a book club and church group. A friend, Norma, who lives across the street, joins her in these activities. Irene, ever the modern senior, owns and uses a computer for E-mail and paying some of her bills on-line.

Irene's philosophy of living arrangements and future plans are well known to her children. She has no intention of living with anyone should she become incapacitated. Her intent is to proceed to assisted living or skilled nursing if her health requires this because she is very social and, at this point, does not think she ever wants to live with her children.

Two Philosophies

These two individuals represent not so much different philosophies as they do two different personality types. Ardelle's preference to lead a private life is not new to her. For example, growing up in the country, she had never driven a car, something that was not an uncommon situation during the years when she was first married. She had remained insecure about learning to drive and never did so even when encouraged by John in later years. John had taken care of most business matters while she had preferred to place her focus on taking care of her home and family. Irene, in contrast, had grown up in the city, always displaying an independent personality. Her family had encouraged her to work at a young age. She had driven a car all her life and worked at her own job for many years before her husband retired.

In summary, the personalities that these two women had displayed during their early years were still at work in their later years. Any attempts to change them now would be a daunting task indeed. These examples illustrate that there is more than one successful living arrangement in later life and that personality is a major consideration when making these plans. The current success of these two individuals in falls prevention is owing to different reasons. In Ardelle's case, her living with her family allowed closer supervision of her activities and greater attention to safety features in her environment. Moving with her husband at an earlier age when she was still able to make the adjustment quite easily probably added several years of independence. Irene, in contrast, has not had severe falls, owing perhaps to her greater level of physical activity over her life span. However, her future in regard to falls is uncertain. Being extremely independent may cause her to not report falls until a major injury occurs. Closer monitoring by the family is warranted at this point in see that safety features are installed and that her activities are carried out in as safe a manner as possible.

How Are Behaviors Changed?

As already mentioned, modifying the environment for safety is one way of automatically controlling behavior to a great extent. However, some behaviors, such as habitual rushing, performing dangerous maneuvers, or doing two things at once, are conditions that are worth attempting to modify more directly.

When someone is in their nineties, standing on a step stool without handles, rushing to answer the telephone or the doorbell, or taking long walks alone at night is not wise behavior, yet such activities are frequently engaged in by older or fall-prone individuals. This may be out of habit, deteriorating judgment, or a **desire to prove one's capabilities to oneself**. Whatever the reason, these activities are all too common and are often participated in with the complete knowledge of the risks and consequences. On the positive side, it is our experience that **changing unwise or risky behaviors is often possible and is one of the most effective means of preventing falls**.

Behavior modification is a popular and sometimes effective way to change a person's behavior. This theory, used by many psychologists, is based on the premise that analyzing the patient's past or subconscious is not as important as trying to change the patient's current thinking and behavior. The system is a positive one, based mainly on rewards, encouragement, and reinforcing positive behavior until a new habit is achieved. Criticism is used minimally and is looked on as largely detrimental to the patient's self-esteem, which is an important element for the patient to have when a new goal is being worked on. Some interesting past findings relating to these principles are discussed in articles by Kirkhart, Robert, and Evelyn (1972) and Gottman and Levenson, (1999).

Aaron Beck, M.D., taught in the 1970s that a person's thoughts are a primary point of intervention and that if assumptions, core beliefs, and automatic thoughts are changed, changes in emotions and behaviors would also occur.

It is well known in the medical community that simply lecturing or "educating" is not an effective way to bring about change. Lecturing is specifically known to be ineffective in preventing falls. It is more effective to help the patient arrive at his or her own conclusions regarding the problem as well as the solutions. Getting this to happen is challenging and time consuming, yet well worth the effort. The following are key elements we have found to be effective in bringing about these changes.

1. Identify habits that are increasing risk of falls by learning about the patient's daily and weekly activities as well as the floor plan of the living environment.
2. Try to help the patient and family to determine why he or she is engaging in the risky, fall-prone behavior.
3. During counseling with the help of family or friends, help the patient to arrive at possible alternatives to dangerous fall-inducing activities.

Other Methods

The principles upon which the above techniques are based are influenced by current established counseling principles. In **psychoeducational counseling**, information about the patient's medical condition is combined with an exploration of the feelings and values of the patient. For example, some of the newer behavior changing techniques are showcased in the media by popular television "psychotherapists." These "half-hour instant personality makeovers" are rough, condensed versions of more recognized techniques carried out by bona fide therapists during long-term therapy. Once the "client" has expressed frustration and dissatisfaction with the current situation, the question is asked what he or she currently does to solve the problem. The person responds by relating his or her own less-than-adequate solution. The person is then asked the key confrontational question, which is something along the lines of,

"How's that working for you?"

"Not well" is the usual response.

At this point, the error of the client's ways are pointed out after which the question is asked,

"What do you think a better solution to this problem might be?"

The client, one hopes, then comes up with his or her own solution. In actual falls clinic counseling situations, the process is aided by the input of friends, family, and the clinician to help the patient arrive at solutions. It is important to keep in mind that the patient's own belief in the solution is very important (Gordon & Duffy, 1998).

The reader is also referred to other current techniques which may prove useful in the falls prevention setting. These include:

1. **Behavioral counseling**, in which the patient is involved in self-assessment and reporting (DiMatteo, 1991).
2. **Motivational interviewing** (Miller & Rollnick, 1991).
3. **Social learning**, a refined type of "peer pressure" (Aubert, Herman, Waler, et al., 1998; Bandura, 1986; Schwazzer, 1992).

Researchers have studied measures that medical personnel can take to change behaviors. For example, "prevention counseling" has been studied in the medical setting, showing that it is important for measures beyond the office visit be taken for the counseling to be effective. Studies show that a proper infrastructure can be set up to support the counseling after the office visit, including involving the office staff, setting up reminder systems, offering appropriate referrals, developing a network of role models, and arranging adequate follow-up (Department of Health and Human Services Public Health Service, Office of Disease Prevention and Health Promotion, 1994; Woolf, Jonas, & Lawrence, 1995).

Office staff should be nonjudgmental, positive, and supportive of the patient even when there is evidence of noncompliance with recommendations (Vogt & Kapp, 1987).

In our clinic, we have effectively used phone calls after the visit to remind patients of their goal, no falls.

Do Behaviors Really Cause Falls?

To further illustrate how falling is largely a behavioral issue, think about this hypothetical, although unrealistic, example. Consider the extreme situation in which a patient never leaves a wheelchair, falling seldom if ever occurs. Someone could chose to never leave a wheelchair even though capable (we are not recommending this). Just for illustration, let us continue the logic to the next level of freedom. If the patient only left a wheelchair when there was some stable individual to hold onto, there would still be very little chance of falling, but some chance. Proceeding to the next degree of freedom, what would happen if a slightly greater element of risk were added, such as when a patient moves about while keeping the wheelchair close at hand in case he or she needs to sit? You may be realizing at this point that all along this continuum of independence, elements of the patient's personality combined with the medical condition come into play. But behavioral issues often rule the day. Is the person the least bit daring? Is he an inherent "risk taker?" The more daring the person, the greater the risk will be. Going to the opposite extreme, if a fall-prone person were to be walking unassisted in dark unfamiliar territory, it would be a very risky behavior, but it may be considered "worth the risk" to many fall-prone individuals. As you can see, short of just sitting in a chair all the time, the **behavioral factors are very relevant**. Sometimes the behavioral factors are the only things that can be modified. If falling is already occurring, there are usually some bad habits, risky or reckless behaviors or at least some wrong mobility techniques occurring. We observe in our clinic that frequent fallers often are persons having a "fall-prone" personality (i.e., those who have a tendency to rush or take chances they know are dangerous). Such persons perform dangerous acts such as using ladders even when they know the risks involved. This type of behavior often goes on in secret. Dangerous behaviors such as using a step stool can be more frequent when the patient is home alone because the chance of being "caught" and chastised is lower.

But what can be done for people who insist on taking chances? It is well known that lecturing or counseling in the aging population has little effect. Changing a bad habit established over a lifetime is even more difficult. It is said that we spend a lifetime perfecting our faults!

Replacing Old Habits with New

The concept of trading old habits for new ones is not new. The problem is, this is easier said than done for two reasons. First, the bad habit is already in place, whereas the new habit to replace it is not yet ingrained. Second, the bad habit is usually enjoyable to a certain extent, whereas the new habit may be too ambitious or not perceived as enjoyable. For example, if one is trying to replace the bad habit of smoking with the good habit of exercising, this may fail due to the fact that smoking is something the person enjoys, whereas the new habit or exercise is not yet enjoyable. But smoking is an extreme example of a habit that is very difficult to break. It involves not only behavioral aspects but bodily cravings as well; therefore, ideas such as simply chewing gum or sucking on candy is less successful because the gum (unless it is nicotine gum) or candy does not fulfill all the bodily cravings that smoking does. But the risky habits we are talking about in this book are not quite the same. Standing on a dangerous step stool or using the stairs improperly may indeed be a habit, but they are not even in the same league as smoking in terms of difficulty in breaking the habit and replacing it with a new one. Step stools are usually not so enjoyable or addicting. Some "new habit" examples relating to falls safety are shown in Table 6-1. Hopefully, the new habits will be even more enjoyable than the dangerous old habits. For example, carrying clothes down the stairs is very dangerous, and not much fun. But throwing dirty clothes down the stairs could possibly be

Table 6–1. Safe and Enjoyable "New Habits" for Falls Prevention

New Habit	Old Habit
Use a long-handled "grabber"	Reaching up or using a stool
Install a "clapper" for lights	Walking in the dark to find the light switch
When getting up at night, hold onto something while saying a poem or prayer before walking	Jumping up and feeling dizzy
Place soap in the soap holder in the shower avoids a slippery floor	Having to pick up the soap
Have a flashlight by the bed	Searching for a flashlight
Carrying a portable phone	Having to go and find the phone
Throw dirty clothes down the stairs	Carrying things on stairs makes holding on more difficult
Use bedside urinal	Rushing to bathroom at night
Take the walker or shopping cart or a friend	Walking too far unassisted
Find the sidewalk	Walking on soft surfaces
Practice "Safe-Walk"	Walking or turning too quickly

more fun and is certainly a lot safer. Using a long-handled "grabber" makes reaching items that are too high, much easier than getting out the step stool and using it. Carrying a portable phone for safety makes it easier to get to the phone than not carrying one.

Safe and Enjoyable "New Habits" for Falls Prevention

As seen in Table 6-1, if new habits are made to be more enjoyable than old ones, they will be more easily accepted.

Older individuals are very interested in learning new things and enjoy the added attention that learning situations often bring.

The philosophy of our Falls Prevention Clinic is to **teach new skills rather than trying to break old habits**. New ways of walking or turning, reaching skills, and other safety-centered habits are welcomed information and skills that can be easily learned.

Let us look at some common bad habits to explore why these habits are so dangerous.

Bad Habit: Reaching Up

Reaching up and tipping the head back is dangerous for several reasons.

1. When the head tilts back, the inner ear is placed in a "dizzy prone" position, which can within a few seconds lead to vertigo in many people with "benign positional vertigo." This common disorder may be present to varying degrees in a high percentage of older individuals.
2. Tilting the head back strains the neck in two ways that can cause dizziness. Nerves in the neck leading to the balance system can be stimulated causing "cervical vertigo." Also, blood vessels in the back of the neck (vertebral and basilar arteries) can be pinched off leading to a decreased blood flow to the head. This results in lightheadedness or even fainting.
3. Reaching up is also dangerous because it causes the body to arch backward, which in the extreme case, requires a quick step backward to catch oneself. Such quickness is often lacking in the aged causing a backward fall.
4. Finally, reaching up keeps one hand busy instead of holding on.

Bad Habit: Doing Two Things at Once

Walking and keeping our balance without falling requires more conscious effort the older we get. Doing two things at once divides our attention and distracts us. This is true at any age. Driving, for example, while fiddling with the telephone or CD player has led to many accidents. Walking while writing, reading, or looking at something in our hands can lead to trips or near falls at any age, but with younger people, such trips or near falls are easily recoverable because quick adjustments of the legs are still possible. In older people, however, such adjustments are slower and often not quick enough to prevent us from toppling over. Carrying something on the stairs is particularly dangerous because, for one thing, this prevents us from holding onto the rail.

Bad Habit: Walking Outside the Home at Night Alone

At least two times of life are dangerous periods for walking outside at night, childhood and old age. The reasons are the same, however. As our mother used to say, there are "things" or situations out there that are dangerous and the individual in trouble may be incapable of getting himself out of that trouble. At night there are generally fewer people to help us out, less light by which to see the ground, and if we do fall it is harder for someone else to find us because it is dark.

Bad Habit: Bending Over Forward (especially on soft surfaces)

Just as reaching upward leads to falls, bending forward, especially on soft ground such as grass or dirt, often leads to falls. The head-down position adversely stimulates the inner ear balance centers as well as the neck nerves leading to balance centers in the brainstem. Also, blood may rush to our head causing a change in blood pressure. Our center of gravity, when bending far forward, makes a forward fall imminent unless the legs are ready to supply a sudden forward movement to catch ourselves.

Bad Habit: Rushing (walking or turning too quickly)

Moving about quickly lends itself to more accidents. In addition, the turning movement is a particularly disturbing stimulation to the inner ear balance mechanism. Fluid in the semicircular canals is displaced with rotational head acceleration in any plane. This may elicit the "benign positional vertigo." Also, head movement such as when rushing, may cause blurred visual perception (oscillopsia). Oscillopsia is a failure of the eyes to reflexively move in the direction opposite to the head movement (a natural reaction of the vestibular-ocular reflex [VOR]). This reflex keeps our visual target on the center of the retina by moving the eyes automatically in the opposite direction of the body's movement. A person with this problem may have a variety of uncompensated inner ear disorders causing him to complain that "things that I am looking at jiggle when I walk." Or "words on signs are blurry when I walk."

"SafeWalk"
A Walking Technique for Falls Prevention

People hate to be told what they are not supposed to do but people of any age welcome the opportunity to learn something new. After interviewing hundreds of fallers in our clinic, it is apparent that even when there are significant medical reasons for falls, many if not most falls occur when people are pushing the limits of their capabilities. Rushing, walking too far unassisted, walking in darkened rooms, walking on soft surfaces such as lawn or sand, carrying something on stairs, or getting up quickly without holding onto something are some of the typical scenarios surrounding most falls we hear about. Simply **turning too quickly** while walking is a simple action that often leads to falls. Practicing the "safe turning method" portion of the SafeWalk techniques explained below helps to eliminate falls stemming from turning too quickly while walking. The old adage may be true, "we spend a lifetime perfecting our faults." At least it is true that old habits developed over a lifetime are hard to break; but in our experience you can teach new habits more easily than break old ones.

Elderly people especially love the attention of being taught how to do new things. Notice in the example in Table 6-1, rushing to the bathroom, that the solution involves doing something new, that is, developing a new habit such as using a bedside commode, whereas other solutions, such as not drinking before bed, involve not doing something that is already a habit (breaking an old habit). Beginning a new habit is easier than breaking an old one, so the better choice would be to start using a bedside commode. Of course, individual differences will influence the decision. Most solutions in Table 6-1 involve the positive approach of doing something new with the hoped for outcome of developing new habits.

Elements of "SafeWalk"

Instability while walking, although dangerous in and of itself, is made much worse by several bad habits especially during certain phases of the walking pattern. Such factors can be controlled to a great extent by learning new walking techniques. SafeWalk employs the elements of slowing down, having nothing in the hands, stopping before turns and turning at the trunk, waiting to walk after first standing, and not walking in the dark (Figure 6-1).

People resist being told what they are not supposed to be doing but are often more receptive to learning a new behavior. People of all ages often love learning something new and elderly people especially love the attention of being taught how to do something different. Notice in the example in Table 6-1, rushing to the bathroom, that the solution involves *doing something new, that is*, **developing a new habit** such as using a bedside commode, whereas other solutions, such as not drinking before bed, involve *not doing something* that is already a habit (**breaking an old habit**). At an advanced age, **beginning a new habit makes it**

SAFEWALK ELEMENTS

Walking slowly

Having nothing in the hands

Stopping before turns and turning at the trunk

Waiting to walk after first standing

Not walking in darkened areas

Not rushing

Not doing more than one thing at once (being distracted while walking)

Not beginning to walk immediately after standing

Walking only where there is light

Figure 6-1. SafeWalk elements for patients.

easier to replace an old habit. Of course, individual differences will influence the decision. Most solutions in Table 6–1, involve the more positive approach of doing something new thereby developing new habits. "SafeWalk" utilizes this philosophy to help a balance-impaired individual replace an unsafe walking style with a new safer one. The old style the individual is using may not always have been unsafe; in fact, it may be normal for persons without impaired balance, but the decrease in balance ability requires a safer style of walking.

Try standing on one leg and you will see that balance is, of course, much more difficult. But when we turn while walking we are actually momentarily standing on one leg for a portion of a second. The "**safe turning method**" means turning the upper body before moving the feet in a new direction. When we turn quickly while walking, we are actually standing on one foot in the middle of a turn. This may be easy for an unimpaired or younger person but it is much more dangerous for an older person or person with impaired balance. Turning the body first, while leaving the feet planted and then moving the feet, is a fun "new" way of turning that an older person is very willing to learn and practice. Even the act of paying attention to the way we walk while practicing helps to reduce falls.

Another fun habit that prevents falls due to standing up quickly and walking too soon while lightheaded, is to recite a short poem before taking a step.

Medical Intervention

Medical intervention is the most straightforward solution to falls prevention. Although a simple medical solution is sometimes not attainable due to the patient having multifactorial causes of falls, many patients do have a primary medical cause of their falling even though it would seem that age alone or the sum total of their medical problems accounts for their falling. The first duty of the clinician is to seek a **main medical cause** for falling even among those who would seem to have a multifactorial cause of falls. For example, many otherwise sick individuals still have coexisting BPPV, peripheral neuropathy, or another distinct entity, without which they would not yet be fallers. Discovering these distinct entities requires a systematic approach as outlined in Chapter 5 on the Falls Examination; however, the clinician should keep in mind that, most often, a medical solution will not be found to the problem of falling. Especially those having degenerative disease, deteriorating strength, or extreme advancing age will not have a single distinct medical entity causing their falls. Although a few patients fortunately are easily "cured" of their falling disorder, sadly the cause of many patients' falls is multifactorial. Still, falls may be prevented in this group through behavioral changes, use of appropriate equipment, and protective strategies. Simply attempting to apply a medical model for "curing" fallers often leads to a long road of endless tests. One of the main roles of a falls clinic is to provide solutions along the way, even when the patient's final diagnosis has not yet been attained.

Canalyth Repositioning (Epley Maneuver, etc.)

One very common medical condition that often can lead to falls is benign paroxysmal positional vertigo (BPPV). Luckily, this disorder is easily treatable by "repositioning maneuvers" performed in the office. These maneuvers are aimed at repositioning crystals, of calcium carbonate back into their normal area of the inner ear anatomy. These procedures are painless and usually effective. Audiologists as well as physical therapists and some physicians perform the procedure. There is much current information about the topic of BPPV as well as the maneuvers for its remediation. Patients often are discovered to have the cardinal sign of BPPV, a positive Dix-Hallpike sign, which is eye jerking when the head is placed back 45 degrees below supine and the head turned to either side 45 degrees. There are many excellent current texts and articles on the topic of BPPV, the Hallpike test, and the canalyth repositioning maneuvers. The reader is referred to the Internet where many excellent articles are most easily obtained.

Vestibular Rehabilitation

Another common inner ear disorder, uncompensated vestibulopathy, which is most often due to a previous episode of vestibular neuritis, is effectively treated with exercises the patient performs involving head movements while fixating the eyes on various targets. The cardinal sign of uncompensated vestibulopathy is a positive head shake test, in which head shaking while vision is denied produces nystagmus immediately afterward. Audiologists and physical therapists are the professionals most often trained in vestibular rehabilitation. Again, the reader is referred to the Internet for current articles on this subject.

Counseling

In our experience, patients are agents unto themselves; that is, unless there is a case of mental incapacity, no one but the patient can make certain that recommendations will be carried out. Prescriptions or recommendations may be given with the patient nodding agreement, but actual compliance is often less than desired; therefore, thought should be given regarding how the clinician may most effectively influence the future actions of the patient and family. In this regard, we have found it most effective to determine one or two "main causes" of falls and then focus the counseling on these areas of change. Other suggestions and recommendations can be furnished later in the final report. Only so much time can be spent individually with the patient and it is more productive to spend that time helping the patient come to his or her own conclusion about the cause of falls. This philosophy argues against calling the patient's cause of falls "multifactorial." It is better to focus the counseling efforts on one or two "main causes" rather than trying to solve all the patient's falls risk factors. The solution must be agreeable to the patient or nothing is accomplished. The goal of the counseling is to have the patient agree to some solution even if that solution is not the first choice of the clinician. A patient recently seen in our clinic had the common problem of sometimes falling when rushing to the bathroom at night. Trips to the bathroom at night are always more dangerous due to less light, a lower level of mental alertness, as well as whatever medical problem is going on. This case could have been considered "multifactorial," as it indeed was, in that a combination of factors were present including orthostatic hypotension causing lightheadedness on rising, a balance disorder of probable central cause, urinary problems causing incontinence, and the behavioral issue of rushing to avoid soiling clothes or bed. In this case, there were several ways of solving the falls problem including use of a bedside commode, not drinking water past 5 o'clock at night, and finding solutions to the medical problems. The question was, which if any of these would the patient actually do? It was decided that the main cause of falls would be considered the trips to the bathroom at night. The remainder of our time was spent focusing on how the patient could avoid these nightly trips to the bathroom. Medical solutions were already being looked into, but having the patient avoid drinking water would serve to worsen her hypotension. On further inquiry, it was discovered that a bedside commode would be acceptable to the patient, but it was not possible due to the extremely small size of her room which would not accommodate even something that small beside her bed. The room was actually a sort of den near the front door of her son's house in which she was living. She had chosen to live in this room because, in the early months of her living there she was often left alone at night and she wanted to be close to the front door so that she could hear any intruder coming in. The son no longer was away from home and so it was determined by the family that changing her room to a larger one would now be acceptable to her and could accommodate the commode. This is an example of how a nonmedical solution is often most practical in the short run, at least while medical issues are being settled. It is also an example of how behavioral issues are usually at the heart of falls prevention.

Role of the "Falls Clinic" in Preventing Falls

The Falls Clinic's role in preventing falls is to identify medical causes of falls, recommend a plan for instituting behavioral changes, and recommend environmental modifications that lower the risk falls and injury for a particular individual. Quite often, the Falls Team helps the individual, along with family if possible, to arrive at living quarters changes that sometimes result in the individual deciding to move to safer surroundings, modify daily or weekly routines, or change the manner in which activities are performed. Switching bedrooms, shopping at a store with heavier shopping carts or motorized carts, having grab bars or other safety features installed are all decisions that occur in the final meeting portion of the clinic visit.

Preventing falls is an individualized effort; that is, what may help one person may not help another. For example, for people who do not have a falling problem, having a great deal of furniture may increase falls risk because there is more to stumble over. However, for "frequent fallers," having lots of furniture is very helpful because these items give the patient something to hold onto as he or she walks or to fall up against. Exercise is also something that can benefit one individual but increase the risk of falls in another. Therefore, falls prevention strategies are very individualized plans that must be formulated for the person and his or her living situation. An individualized falls prevention plan (IFP) should be provided to the patient at the end of the Falls Clinic visit.

Patient Accountability

Accountability is an important aspect of the falls prevention plan. In our experience, advising the patient that he or she will be called in a few weeks to ask for a report on progress is an important aspect of the follow-up. If posturography is used and improvement in balance score is very likely, asking the person to return in a period of 2 to 6 months to retake the test to demonstrate improvement of the balance score is an extremely motivating activity. If there is improvement in the score, this is even more motivating.

Stress the Positive

Being positive about the results of tests during the falls clinic visit, by emphasizing the patient's strengths, is extremely important. When analyzing the results of balance tests on older individuals, it is easy to see the "glass half empty" due to the characteristic poor balance of most aging individuals. This can be a very discouraging report, but it should not be. Emphasizing the individual's strong points goes much further toward eliciting cooperation than dwelling on all of the patient's deficits. As bad as the balance situation may be, a great deal of improvement usually can be achieved if the patient is motivated. By stressing the positive and setting forth realistic expectations, reduction or elimination of falls is generally achievable with most patients.

Nutrition

Vitamin D has been implicated in helping to reduce falls due to its positive effects on musculoskeletal function.

Postprandial orthostatic hypotension may occur, which is a 20 mmHg drop in systolic blood pressure within 2 hours of a meal.

Exercise

Exercise is a "two-edged sword" in falls prevention. Although there is no doubt that the known benefits of exercise also are helpful in reducing falls, there are studies which show that, in many persons, exercising leads to more falls because more situations occur in which the patent is not holding onto something. The point is, exercise is helpful but it also must be safe. "Safe" exercise essentially consists of exercising while holding onto something. Of course, standard exercise equipment comes to mind such as a stationary bicycle or treadmill but then the patient is not practicing normal walking. Also, we may picture exercising while holding onto a handrail, which also may limit the type of exercise that may be performed. One of the best exercises we have found is walking behind a shopping cart. Stable large shopping carts found in large hardware stores or supermarkets provide a safe support for most elderly fallers. Scouting the route in advance is important to ensure that there are an adequate number of rest areas such as chairs or benches. Having someone accompany the person is also a good idea.

Exercising in a swimming pool can overcome the challenges faced by individuals who are weak or extremely overweight.

The pros and cons of exercise of various types have been studied; however, the data are conflicting at this point. Therefore, we will not review these studies, believing instead in the common sense conclusion that safe exercise is beneficial for reducing falls risk in most persons. One exercise that repeatedly shows up in studies as beneficial is Tai Chi. It is not known exactly why this particular exercise is helpful but considering its style, it is easy to speculate the reasons. Tai Chi involves keeping the legs and feet stationary most of the time, which allows for stable safe support. On the other hand, the arms and head are moved in a slow circular dancelike fashion, which appears to be both stimulating and challenging to the balance system, particularly the vestibular system (semicircular canals and related structures). The movements of Tai Chi seem to resemble those recommended in vestibular rehabilitation exercises, in which the eyes are coordinated with head movements to recalibrate the vestibular-ocular and other reflexes associated with the vestibular system.

Evaluating and Modifying Living Areas

Evaluating the patient's living environment is key to preventing falls; however, this section asserts that behaviors related to a patient's environment are even more critical. Only by assessing the patient's behaviors in relation to the environment will falls prevention be maximized.

There are several ways to evaluate a person's living environment for falls risk. These include on-site inspections, clinic-based interviews given in person, or written questionnaires. On-site inspections are favored by physical or occupational therapists because they appreciate the fact that items may be forgotten by the patient when trying to fill out a questionnaire or respond to questions. Also, being on site allows the therapist to better make specific recommendations regarding the space and its contents. Such visits may be expensive, and therefore impractical, although they may be made by certain insurances especially when the patient is considered "home bound." Some community based "falls prevention programs" are based solely on these in-home evaluations. Next best would probably be the one-on-one interview in the clinic. Asking questions in person allows for immediate clarification and discussion in which suggestions may be made and solutions offered. We often make a rough sketch of the floor plan of the home with the help of the patient. This helps the examiner to visualize the floor plan better and determine where grab bars or other safety features may be most effectively installed.

It is best to approach the subject of home safety features with an emphasis on behavior. It is really the person's habits and behavior in relation to the environment that matter most. For example, during the discussion with one recent patient, a risky situation was identified. The patient was carrying grocery items into the home using outside stairs that did not have a handrail. By sketching out the floor plan, identifying the locations of steps leading to the outside, it was determined that there were three sets of steps, at the front, back, and side of the house, all leading inside. The only steps without a handrail were those at the side of the house leading directly into the family room. Those were the steps being used to carry in groceries because that route provided the shortest distance to the kitchen by a small amount. It was determined that, although the back steps would mean having to carry the groceries a few steps farther, it would be far safer to use those steps for carrying in groceries because they contained a handrail. However, the act of carrying groceries was also risky. The patient came up with the solution herself of putting the groceries into a small wheeled cart which she already owned and using that to transport the groceries to the back steps. The cart would carry more groceries than could be carried by hand, so now the new safer solution would also be the easier one.

Evaluation of the patient's living quarters is important on several levels. Although the living environment can almost always be improved in terms of reducing hazards or adding safety features, there are broader considerations for the patient's living environment respecting falls risk. When discussing the living environment with the patient, it should be remembered that this is where the person spends most of his or her time; therefore, the patient's daily habits relate in a major way to this discussion. For example, when discussing the kitchen, it is important to discuss not only where obstacles are, but also the patient's activities in that room. In fact, the questions asked should stress more the behavior involved than the obstacle itself. For example, does the patient spend considerable time standing while cooking? Could a stool be employed while cooking to reduce falls risk? Are trips made to the kitchen at night when there is less light? Is there extra lighting available or can this be installed?

Using behavior-related questions is far more effective than simply applying a checklist of home safety features. Some items in the home are more risky under certain circumstances. For example, stairs are much more dangerous in the dark, especially for persons who rely more on their visual balance such as those with vestibular problems. Others who have more problems in the dark include those who have reduced feeling in the feet and, therefore, rely more heavily on their sense of vision for balance.

The following list (Figure 6–2) consists of **behavior-based questions** to be considered when evaluating the living environment either on site or by interview in the clinic. In the section following the questions, more detailed information about the questions is provided.

Evaluation of the Living Environment
"Behavior Based" Questions

Living Room: Yes   No

Do you ever get up and rush to answer the door?   ☐   ☐

Do you ever get up and rush to answer the telephone?   ☐   ☐

Do you live with other people who can help you if you fall?   ☐   ☐

Are the people who live with you aware of the importance
of reducing clutter on floors?   ☐   ☐

Which doors do you use leading to the outside the house?   ☐   ☐

Are you ever confused as to where one of the doors leads?   ☐   ☐

If a door leads to stairs, is there a handrail on all steps
within or outside of the house?   ☐   ☐

Could you place additional items of furniture in your living
room to hold onto?   ☐   ☐

Are there coffee or couch tables that could be dangerous?
Could you trip over these or might you hurt yourself if you
were to fall onto them (glass or breakable wood).   ☐   ☐

Bathroom:

Do you get up in the night to use the bathroom?   ☐   ☐

Do you take showers or baths? _____

Do you have trouble getting into or out of the tub or shower?   ☐   ☐

Is there a chair or stool in the shower or tub?   ☐   ☐

Do you put the soap back into the soap dish after using it?   ☐   ☐

Do you use safety mats in the shower or tub?   ☐   ☐

Do you feel faint or dizzy after getting up from using
the toilet?   ☐   ☐

Would you consider using a raised toilet seat and/or
handles to the sides of the toilet?   ☐   ☐

Figure 6–2. Evaluation of the living environment *continues*

Bedroom:	Yes	No
Do you get up in the night to go to the bathroom?	☐	☐
Would a bedside commode make going to the bathroom safer for you?	☐	☐
Do you drink a "night cap" before going to bed or take sleeping or pain pills?	☐	☐
Are there night-lights on so that you can see the floor when getting up?	☐	☐
Do you need a flashlight by your bed in case the lights go out?	☐	☐

Kitchen:

What door do you use to carry in groceries? Are there rails on the steps leading in? _____

	Yes	No
Do you stand very long while cooking?	☐	☐
Would using a stool for cooking make you less likely to fall?	☐	☐
Do you have to carry your food from the cooking area to a separate table?	☐	☐
Would it help you to have items placed lower in cupboards so that you don't have to reach up? (this makes many people dizzy)	☐	☐

Stairs:

	Yes	No
Do you use the stairs?	☐	☐
Do you carry things on the stairs? What? _____	☐	☐
Could you use a soft cloth shoulder bag for carrying things instead of carrying them in your hands (which makes it more difficult to hold onto the stairs)?	☐	☐
Could you throw things such as clothing down the stairs to avoid carrying them?	☐	☐
Would if be safer if you took one step at a time?	☐	☐
Do you keep your hand on the rail, sliding it rather than lifting your hand with each step?	☐	☐

Figure 6–2. *continues*

	Yes	No
Do you lead with your strong foot going up and with your weak foot coming down the stairs? (this is usually safest)	☐	☐
Are you ever distracted while using the stairs (talking on the phone or reading something)? This is unsafe.	☐	☐

Out of Doors:

	Yes	No
Do you fall, trip, or nearly fall when entering or leaving the house?	☐	☐
Are there rails on all steps outside the house?	☐	☐
If there are areas outside the home where there is a higher or lower level such as with a patio, is there something to hold onto?	☐	☐

What activities or situations occur when you fall or nearly fall out of doors?

_____

	Yes	No
Do you walk alone at night out of door?	☐	☐
Do you carry a phone with you?	☐	☐

General questions:

	Yes	No
Are there different levels of the floor leading from room to room for which there is no rail or sturdy object to hold onto?	☐	☐

What are example situations in your home that cause you to fall or nearly fall? In what rooms?

_____

_____

	Yes	No
Are there area rugs or throw rugs anywhere in your home?	☐	☐
Are there grab bars, not only in the bathroom, but at other strategic locations in the house?	☐	☐
Are there raised thresholds in doorways that could be removed to prevent tripping?	☐	☐

Figure 6–2. _continued_

Living Room

The living room, for all its warmth and friendliness, is one of the most dangerous rooms in the house with a substantial number of falls occurring here. For one thing, this room is often fairly large, usually having an open area where there is nothing to hold onto. Also, there are items here that may be fallen onto, the most notorious of which is the coffee table. Coffee tables or couch tables are particularly risky because they are low to the floor, easily stumbled over, and often made of breakable material that causes further injury due to the resulting sharp edges. When someone falls onto a coffee table, particularly if it is glass, serious injury frequently occurs. Several of our patients have fallen onto or over coffee or couch tables resulting in injuries. Associated with these tables are also "area rugs," a type of throw rug. Throw rugs are high on the list of dangerous items in the home because no matter, how much double-stick tape is used to secure their edges, people still frequently trip over them. Following the philosophy of physical therapists, **there should be no throw rugs in the home of a person who is at risk of falling**.

Another common occurrence in the living room is **rushing to either the door or the phone**. Rushing, itself a dangerous behavior for potential fallers, is also covered in a separate section on behaviors and their modification. Simple solutions to avoid rushing include the use of portable phones that are kept with the person, and simply shouting the phrase, "I'm coming. Please wait, I take a little while."

A good idea to prevent falls in the living room or other large room is to place extra furniture in open areas that can be held onto or fallen against. We hear of many falls that occur in which the patient would have hit the floor if it had not been for strategically placed furniture. Wherever the person is in the house, **there should always be something to hold onto**.

Living rooms are also places where power cords or other items that can be easily tripped over are sometimes found. Automatic lights that turn on at night are sometimes employed in the living room for security. Such a light also lets the person visualize the floor thus helping to prevent falls.

Bathroom

The word bathroom is nearly synonymous with falls. The slippery wet surfaces of tubs and showers are the most likely places for falls;

however, the toilet and the sink are also common falls locations. The following suggestions apply to these locations.

Toilet. After one uses the toilet, at least three things can happen to the person that may result in falls. Positional vertigo resulting from changes in head positions may cause dizziness after standing up. Perhaps even more common is the situation in which a person experiences a drop in blood pressure (orthostatic hypotension) when going from sitting to standing. A third possibility, the Valsalva response, which is the pressurized compression of the thorax and abdomen that occurs when bearing down during defecation, may cause a **vasovagal** response, which results in a sudden drop in blood pressure accompanied by an increase in heart rate and then a subsequent rise in blood pressure. This can result in fainting (syncope) or near syncope that can lead to a fall. A combination of the above reactions may also occur, as is frequently the case in older patients.

A solution to these problems after using the toilet is using a raised toilet seat. A raised toilet seat allows the patient to not have to change position to as great a degree; therefore, the effects of this change are not usually as great. An added but not trivial benefit is that the effort needed to get up is much less. Raised toilet seats come in several varieties. The simplest is a thick plastic piece placed on top of the regular toilet that simply acts as an extension of the seat itself. Provided that it can be secured to not fall off frequently, this solution is adequate. Separate handles for the toilet can be purchased. A more complex raised toilet seat resembles a walker that is over the toilet with handles on the sides to help the patient get up as well as a separate toilet seat that sits above the original toilet. Advantages of this type are that some versions can be adapted with a receptacle pan and used beside the bed, or alternatively over the regular toilet when desired.

Sink. Standing at the sink in the bathroom also often results in falls. There are at least two possibilities. The head is often extended upward at the sink such as during shaving or applying eye makeup. This head extension can cause vertigo in those who have benign positional vertigo. A partial blockage of a neck artery such as in basilar artery insufficiency may cause faintness or dizziness. Also, cervicogenic or "neck-induced" vertigo may cause nerves in and around the cervical vertebrae or muscles to generate signals to the vestibular system resulting in mild dizziness.

The sink is a place where, after standing for a long time, an elderly person may become weak tending to fall backward. Use of a stool at the sink may prevent falls in this case. Also, we are sometimes distracted doing something at the sink. If an older individual has a weakened sense of balance, such as in bilaterally reduced vestibular response, as is often the case, there is less of a sensation of tipping. In that case, being distracted results in a fall backward before the person is aware of tipping.

Tub or Shower. The bathtub obviously is a dangerous place due to the slippery and wet surfaces. However, bathtubs are also dangerous in that they are difficult to get out of at all for some older or otherwise incapacitated individuals. Many a "long lie" has occurred in which an elderly individual, being alone, has been found in the bathtub a day or more later unable to lift himself or herself out due to generalized weakness sometimes combined with obesity. A fall may have also occurred causing injury that made it more difficult to get out. For these reasons, showers are preferred over bathtubs in fall-prone individuals. There does exist, however, expensive equipment to help lower or raise a person to and from the tub. But, in general, showers can be accessed more easily as well as more easily accommodate a sturdy stool or chair. An extension on the shower head can also make bathing in the shower easier. If only a tub exists, a sturdy stool can still be used in the tub. A flexible extension for the shower head can also be effective in the tub. In either case, there should be a soap holder to keep soap off the floor.

Grab Bars. Grab bars must be sturdy and able to hold the full weight of a falling person. Towel holders are often used but are not adequate for this purpose. A good grab bar should be solidly anchored to the framework of the house, not simply attached with anchors mounted into sheetrock. Grab bars are important at strategic locations to aid in entering or leaving the tub or shower area. It is also a good idea to have a grab bar placed on the outside of the shower area that can be used not only when getting into the shower or tub, but also after leaving these areas. Bending over to dry oneself is an activity leading to falls. A solution is to place something to sit on outside the shower area.

Bedroom

The main risk for falls in the bedroom occurs during the night in the dark. Most elderly patients visit the bathroom one or more times per night. A bedside commode, the best solution in terms of falls prevention, is often frowned on by the patient for obvious reasons. Getting up quickly to go to the bathroom at night is a "triple threat" in that three risk factors are present: darkness, rushing to make the bathroom on time to avoid soiling sheets or clothing, and getting up quickly, as described above. The common problems of BPPV and orthostasis often cause dizziness when rising suddenly, thus complicating an otherwise safe trip to the bathroom. The bedside commode should be stressed when there is a need to rush because the suggestion to wait when standing up before walking most often will be ignored. Alcohol consumption, which many seniors indulge in as a "night cap" to relax before sleeping, further complicates the situation in that there may now be a decrease in balance due to the alcohol. It may be best to ask the patient to devise his or her own solution. First, outline the problems stated above and then ask the patient, "What solution can you come up with to avoid falls that are common in this situation?" A "medical" solution may be preferred, such as may be provided by the primary doctor, which for men, may consist of a treatment or medication for a possible prostate problem. Simply not drinking after about 5:00 PM is a solution frequently offered by the physician. If a medical solution is not forthcoming, the safety precautions should consist of night lights, having something to hold onto such as furniture, holding onto the bed for a minute or two until the dizziness goes away, or reciting a poem or prayer before walking, thus allowing enough time for the balance system to equilibrate (in this dangerous situation, the prayer may be especially needed). Owing to occasional power outages, there is need for a flashlight by the bed. In case of a fall, a portable phone or other alerting device is also a wise addition.

Kitchen

Although it is not thought of as a particularly dangerous room for falling, many falls occur in the kitchen, probably because so much time is spent there and most of it is spent standing or walking. The kitchen is a room to keep a falling person out of if possible;

however, this is seldom practical. Many of the activities involved in cooking require the use of two hands. With both hands occupied, we cannot hold onto something at the same time. For most people, even cracking an egg requires two hands.

Simpler meals are key. If much cooking must be done, microwaving has the advantage of utilizing fewer steps to accomplish. Microwave meals are much improved over those of earlier days, and although not inexpensive, offer good nutrition and a wide variety of choices. Hot entrees for breakfast, lunch, and dinner are available. If sodium content is of concern, the packaging labels may need to be checked as some frozen meals rely heavily on sodium.

Many reported falls in the kitchen occur when coming into or out of the room because there is often a door leading from the kitchen to the outside of the house and falls occur when using that door. This is probably because shopping items are often being carried, thereby increasing the chance of falls or injuries. Carrying things is more dangerous because we are distracted, off-balance due to the weight of the packages, and we do not have our hands as free to balance or catch ourselves if we should fall. The solution, therefore, consists mainly in changing behaviors. In interviewing patients at our clinic, we have learned that many back porch steps do not contain handrails. The lack of something to hold onto is often cited by our patients as the reason for their falls on steps.

Many patients also report falls while standing cooking or washing the dishes. This is probably because many of our patients are elderly and standing for long periods of time increases the chances of falling due to fatigue or, as in the bathroom, not being aware of their tipping because of distractions and a reduced bilateral vestibular input that many of our aging patients have. A tall stool in back of the patient may save the patient from a fall by giving the patient something to fall back on as well as a place for occasional rests.

Carrying food to and from the table also is a risky business. The patient may choose to carry things in the seat of a wheelchair while pushing it from behind if there is adequate ambulation ability.

Reaching up into tall cupboards is also a danger in the kitchen because there is increased tendency to fall backward. Having a vestibular, neck, or other disorder often predisposes the person to dizziness in this head back position.

Having carpeting in the kitchen is a good idea as it acts as padding if a person does fall. Kitchen carpeting is again feasible and quite practical because of the introduction of "carpet tiles." These have recently become popular again as they are less recognizable as tiles because they are better matched. Hotel lobbies and hospital floors often are covered with carpet tiles because each tile can be easily replaced if there are accidents that stain them. Carpet tile sizes are now usually larger than one foot square, but they come in several sizes. Although nylon carpeting is often favored for its quality, polyester has recently been improved. Kitchen carpeting usually will be thinner than that in other areas of the home, but even thin carpeting provides some protection against injury.

Stairs

Most safety lists for falls prevention offer typical suggestions for safety on the stairs, including taking one step at a time, not carrying things if possible, leading with the stronger foot going up and the weaker one coming down (this allows the strong legs to hold its place while the body lowers to the next level), and so forth. One technique that some of our patients have found useful is to go down backward. This is usually safer because going down stairs is somewhat like going down a steep mountain. If you have tried that, you know that it can be terrifying. We do not climb down a steep cliff or mountain facing outward, but rather facing inward toward the mountain. Rapelling is the extreme example, which would be terrifying facing outward. Although climbing down the stairs is not as extreme, still facing inward (going down backward) holding onto the handrail usually with both hands is considered easier by many older people. Climbing down backward is the older individual's way of "rapelling" down the stairs. It is also easier to hold firmly onto the handrail in that position.

In our interviews with many fallers, it has become apparent that **the main problem is the distractions that are occurring while using the stairs**. Whenever we are using the stairs, we are going to do something. We are on our way to someplace where we will be doing the thing that we are probably thinking about at the moment. We are usually anxious to get there and may be talking to someone, looking at something we are holding, or rushing. The following distractions (Table 6-2) should be avoided by anyone who uses stairs.

Table 6–2. Distractions While Using Stairs

Social Interactions	Personal Activities	Environmental
Talking to someone in person	Rushing	Loose carpeting
Talking to someone on the phone	Thinking about what we will be doing soon	Poor lighting
Sending a text message	Worrying about what we just did	Inadequate rails
	Carrying something	Loose steps
	Reading	

Using the stairs is so automatic that we do it without thinking and so we can usually get away with doing something else at the same time such as reading or talking on the phone. Conversations continue on stairs and people sometimes meet and sometimes talk on stairs. The steps leading into churches or other buildings are particularly social places with a lot of greeting and socializing occurring there. For these reasons, many falls are reported on stairs in public places. But stairs in the home are the ones taken more regularly and the distractions encountered there are of our own making. In our "SafeWalk" method, which is a list of new walking habits to prevent falls, the habit suggested is stopping briefly before taking the stairs. This gives our mind a brief moment to realize what it is we are doing. Our mind may think, "Now I'm taking the stairs, so be careful!" Other suggested behaviors on the stairs include, taking one step at a time starting with the same foot on each step. Again, usually the stronger foot leads when going up and the weaker one leads when going down. Keep the hand on the rail, sliding it as you go rather than lifting it each time. This could result in the hand missing the rail on occasion. Review the other suggestions listed in Table 6-2.

In counseling the person who falls on the stairs, it is a good idea to ask the question, "What are you usually doing when you fall?" or "What were you on your way to do when you fell on the stairs?" Very often the patient knows exactly where he or she was going because it is often an occasion out of the ordinary that had a distracting aspect. These questions give the examiner the opportunity of visualizing the situation, thus helping patients to recognize their risky behaviors and arrive at their own solutions. Solutions should include a more specific plan than "just being more careful." The "SafeWalk" technique described above allows a new habit to be formed in the place of an old one.

Distractions—A Major Reason People Fall on Stairs

Although distractions are probably the number one reason people fall on stairs, there are also physical conditions that greatly inhibit normal function on the stairs (Table 6–3). The most common of these include a lack of feeling in the feet (peripheral neuropathy), which often occurs in diabetes and other disorders, visual problems including the use of bifocals or reading glasses which may distort our perception of the distance of our foot from the step, neuromuscular disorders that may cause us not to be able to move our feet as we wish, proprioception disorders (the inability to sense where our foot is without looking), as well as orthopedic problems.

In summary, although falls on stairs may sometimes have a medical basis, distracting behaviors are probably the most common reasons for falls on stairs according to our observations. Focusing

Table 6–3. Health-Related Reasons for Falls on Stairs

Lack of feeling (peripheral neuropathy)
Visual disorders
Use of bifocals
Use of reading glasses on stairs
Motor deficits
Neurological disorder
Proprioceptive disorders

questions on behaviors will allow the clinician the best opportunity to visualize the situation and help the patient arrive at a new behavior.

General Considerations

Door Handles

Generally, handles are easier to hold onto and manipulate safely than are doorknobs. Arthritic hands and fingers can find it difficult to grasp a door knob with sufficient grip to turn it or even hold on safely for support. Door handles are safer in that they can be used as a somewhat stable handle and can be more easily opened.

Legs on Furniture

Legs on furniture can be a hazard when they stick out beyond the borders of the upper surface of the furniture because a foot can be caught on them. On the other hand, legs should be sturdy enough to support the weight of a persons should there be a fall onto the furniture. Furniture that breaks due to weakness in any portion becomes an object having sharp edges that may injure a person who falls on it breaking it.

Night-Lights

Proper lighting has been stressed in this book as an important aid to prevent falls because if there is a decrement in the vestibular or somatosensory balance systems, the visual system must make up the difference. It is estimated that older individuals need nearly 10 times the light that a younger person needs; therefore, simple night-lights are not usually adequate. Lighting needs to be bright enough to display the floor over much of its area, whereas single small-globed night-lights illuminate only a small area around the light. Many options exist to allow for more lighting on the floor including brighter and larger "night-lights," "clapper switches" that can turn on a table lamp or other light, or simply installing a room light switch near the bed. A bathroom light can also be left on all night with the bathroom door cracked open.

Amount of Furniture

The more furniture in the home of a falling individual the better, assuming that the furniture is not low enough to trip over or become a dangerous object if it is broken when fallen against. In that regard, glass doors on buffets or on the front of low cabinets are dangerous as are "coffee tables" or "couch tables" having glass tops or thin wood that may break. Furniture should be at least waist high or it may be tripped over. In summary, having lots of high solid furniture is an advantage to a falling individual for two reasons. The furniture serves as a pathway providing something to hold onto at all locations in the home, and furniture can be fallen against, thus preventing injury.

Carpet

Studies have come to the obvious conclusion that when a person falls on a padded or softer surface, fewer hip fractures occur. Padding either can be worn as in hip pads and other pads or can be in the form of carpeting. Carpeting, if it contains the proper amount of padding, is a very beneficial feature for falls prevention. Carpeting, however, can also cause problems. If the carpeting is too thick, then the leg balance system is at a disadvantage in that the "true flat surface" cannot be detected, particularly if it is dark and vision cannot be utilized. Persons with "inner ear" or vestibular balance system dysfunctions need to rely more heavily on their leg and visual balance systems. Therefore, carpeting can be too thick to be safe in the sense that a person may be more unstable on very thick soft carpeting.

Proper safe carpeting should ideally be of the "plush" or "cut pile" type (also called Saxony or "velvet" although not made of velvet). Carpets that have major disadvantages for falls are shag, frieze, textured, sculptured, or loop pile. These carpets are too dense, bumpier, and often contain small loops that can easily catch on shoes. Carpets of the proper type mentioned above are also good for providing a smooth surface that the foot can more easily slide across. Allowing the foot to slide easily is important for older persons as some have a tendency to shuffle more as they walk. Carpeting having the disadvantages mentioned above makes it more likely for the person with shuffling gait to fall. Carpet thickness should be "cut pile" or "low-cut pile."

"Checklists" for the Home

Although there are several different falls "safety checklists" for the home (see Appendix C), probably of greatest importance in "fall-proofing" the home is a consideration of how the home interacts with individuals at various stages of falls disorders. Measures employed for a high-risk individual who falls often may be different or even the opposite of those employed for an individual with only low risk of falls. For example, those with only small risk of falling may want to remove extra furniture because, being younger and moving about more often in the house, having extra pieces of furniture poses a risk of being obstacles that are in the way. In contrast, very old patients who fall regularly probably would benefit from more pieces of furniture that can be held onto as they navigate slowly from place to place. Such furniture, if not low lying, also serves as something to fall up against or onto when the inevitable falls occur. Therefore, it is wise to consider home modifications separately for differing degrees of fall risk, those who are infrequent fallers, and those who fall regularly.

Home Considerations for "Infrequent Fallers"

Infrequent fallers constitute the largest group of potential fallers and are mainly those who range from being a little unstable when first standing to those who are unstable to varying degrees most of the time, yet still with few falls. The term "few falls" means approximately three falls per year or fewer. Also included in the "infrequent faller" group are those who have occasional but major episodic health events that cause them to fall without warning. For the latter group, the overriding principle for falls protection is that they carry an alerting device of some kind. But for the typical "infrequent faller," although falls occur rarely, they are more likely to fall than people due to some inability to stay balance or move normally. **Safe living space characteristics** for "infrequent fallers" include:

1. **solid, nonslippery walking surfaces**
2. **absence of unexpected hazards** to be tripped over, and
3. **built-in safety features** such as plenty of handrails, grab bars, and special individualized features (bedside commodes, etc.).

A "Fall-Safe Home"

Whether the degree of falls risk is mild or severe ("infrequent" or "frequent"), certain falls prevention guidelines for the home are common to both groups, and actually not a bad idea for the rest of us . The following list (Table 6–4) prioritizes unsafe "fall-prone" physical features of the home in the approximate order of most to

Table 6–4. Unsafe Items in a "Fall-Prone" Home

Throw rugs (even when taped)
Wet surfaces
Slippery surfaces
Handrails absent on stairs, weak, or in need of maintenance
Cupboards or drawer handles in need of maintenance
Absence of grab bars in the bathroom (near toilet, in shower or tub)
Clutter left in unexpected places
Pets underfoot
Legs of furniture that stick out
Absence of night-lights
General absence of adequate lighting
No light switches at top or bottom of stairs
Floors change level abruptly
Objects too high on shelves
Carpet that is too thick
Open areas without something to hold onto
Tub and showers without mats and chairs
Tubs and showers that are difficult to step into
Too few phones
Unusually sticky surfaces
Loose carpet
Soap in shower is loose on floor
No rug outside shower to dry feet
Nonsturdy step stools or ladders
Furniture is hard to get out of
Lack of emergency flashlight

least dangerous. In contrast, Figure 6-3 shows a list of characteristics ideally found in a "Fall-Safe" home. This list is also reproduced as Appendix C in large font for easy photocopying.

Walking Equipment

A walker is extremely helpful for many off-balance patients and can mean the difference between safe and unsafe ambulation. As a simple rule, a walking device should be recommended whenever the patient's gait is observed to be unstable, or when the patient or relative feels a cane or walker is necessary. Of course, many patients have a negative reaction to the idea of a walker. Following are some of the useful ways we have employed to help people accept a walker:

A Walker May Not Need to Be Permanent

A positive approach is best and it is not untruthful to offer hope to many people that their walker may not need to be permanent. The basis for this argument is that a walker allows many more steps per day for many patients than would be taken without one. More steps allows for more exercise, which leads to increased strength and coordination. But not only are strength and coordination increased, there is new evidence that the brain learns to utilize new pathways involving movement when there are repetitive movements occurring even if the normal neural pathways are not functional. Studies involving a new type of therapy termed "repetitive movement therapy" have been performed in animals and humans who have had strokes. When the limb is repetitively moved by either a machine or a therapist in the normal manner, recovery rates are much greater. Apparently the brain assigns new pathways to make up for those lost by the stroke or injury. Such "plasticity" of neural function has been proven for arm movements and is currently being studied for other types of movements. Although plasticity is known to decrease in older individuals, there is still evidence of some plasticity among older people. An example case will help to illustrate the principles just described.

Ted (named changed) was seen in the Falls Clinic after a surgery on his cerebellum, which caused him to lack coordinated movement

CHARACTERISTICS OF A "FALL-SAFE" HOME

Stairways

Install handrails at all stairways
Do the handrails support a person's weight?
Keep floors and steps clear of clutter
Throw away "throw rugs"
Use colored tape at the top and bottom of stairs
to identify the first and last step
Good lighting at all locations in the house,
especially for use at night

Bathroom

Install grab bars near bathtub, shower, and toilet
Keep soap in the soap holder
Place nonslip rubber mats in the bathtub and shower
Nonskid rug outside the bathtub to dry feet
Elevated toilet seats or handles
Bedside commode

Family Room, Bedroom and Kitchen

Wipe up spills
Use floor wax that is slip-resistant.
Wait for floors to dry after cleaning
Avoid cords, oxygen tubing, and
other hazards in pathways
Place commonly used items in easy to reach locations
Do not use stepladders or stools to stand on
(use a long-handled "reacher" or
rearrange objects to lower shelves)
Avoid chairs having wheels
Chairs should have arm rests for easy exiting
When rising, stand slowly if dizziness
occurs, and regain balance before walking
Use automatic on/off night-lights to light pathways
Always keep a charged flashlight and
telephone in your bedrooms for
emergencies
Carry a portable phone or safety alert

Note: The above list is reproduced in large font
as Appendix C for easy photocopying.

Figure 6–3. Characteristics of a "fall–safe" home.

in his legs. He could walk only with great effort, sometimes taking several minutes to move a few feet ahead. If he did not hold onto something or someone he often fell. Ted had recently been "young and active" and was discouraged by his present condition. Being a very determined person, he felt that, in relearning to walk, he should "do it the hard way" to improve faster. He felt that if he were to use a walker his body would learn to depend on the device and not learn to walk as easily. He would be taking the easy way out. After trying a walker in the clinic, it was obvious to Ted as well as the family, that the device allowed him to walk quite easily. The concept of "repetitive movement therapy" was explained to Ted, in that if he were to use a walker he could take a "thousand steps per day" whereas without the walker he could take only a few. The concept of plasticity seemed to appeal to Ted. We explained that children having injuries will often use a walker to progress faster. Without the walker, many such children would remain immobile indefinitely. Such children may then graduate to small leg braces and eventually walk without any assistive device. Ted agreed to use the walker on the basis of his new understanding that the walking aid would be a possible means to improvement.

Of course, many older individuals with deteriorating health may never recover so dramatically by use of a walker, still we never know who may improve and to what extent. At the very least, the walker promotes greater strength and flexibility as well as maintains coordination and cardiovascular exercise. We also feel that it is not unreasonable to offer hope to patients of any age or condition that a walker at the least will lead to some improvement in strength or balance. Such a counseling approach allows the walker to be seen as a rehabilitation tool and not as a sign of deteriorating health.

A Walker May Be the Means of Remaining Independent

The benefits mentioned above—improvement in strength or balance—may or may not occur; however, what is undoubtedly true is that, if a walker is helpful in ambulation, such a device will help to keep the individual independent longer. Therefore, we stress that the walker is not being recommended to punish the patient but to serve as a means of greater happiness and independence for the patient.

Physical therapists prefer a walker with wheels only on the front. This arrangement allows for easy movement, yet prevents the walker from sliding too quickly because the back legs which have no wheels act as brakes whenever the patient stops moving and places weight on the walker. Four-wheeled walkers, which are becoming very popular, have a potential risk of "running away" with the patient or possibly sliding out from under the patient when attempting to sit on the seat that is often attached to the walker. The hand brakes that are made to prevent this problem can be confusing to some patients. These statements, however, are only conjectures by the author and not based on any reliable research at this point.

Canes

Canes can either help or hinder a patient's balance and can, in some people, even increase the risk of falls. Therefore, the patient should be observed while using a cane to see if the gait and stability are improved or not. Just providing a cane or walker is often an ineffective strategy for preventing falls, as there is evidence that, for many individuals, walking aids do not prevent falls. On the negative side, the use of a cane or walker can modify a patient's posture. In the case of a walker, this has been shown in certain individuals to modify "automatic postural responses," which may actually decrease balance ability. Canes can easily become tangled with the patient's legs, thereby increasing falls risk. Four-pronged canes, which increase stability in some individuals, are too heavy for others, thereby decreasing their balance ability. On the positive side, canes can be useful if there is a weakness in one leg relative to the other. Also, a cane is often helpful as an additional "sensor" of the ground, especially for persons who have decreased sensation in the legs or feet. In a sense, the cane serves as another appendage sensing the ground through use of a hand. This allows the patient to sense the horizontal frame of reference as well as detect obstacles or variations in the surface of the ground.

The key to injury prevention when recommending such devices is the judicious use of professional input when choosing the appropriate walking aid so it can be suited to the individual needs of the patient. When recommending walking devices, these should be evaluated by watching the patient use the intended the device so that determination can be made as to appropriateness and type.

Shoes and Footwear

When thinking about appropriate footwear to prevent falls, it should be remembered that we are mainly looking for characteristics that promote good balance. Typical thinking about footwear may not always apply. For example, many people think that athletic shoes would be better for those who may fall because they provide better traction and other aspects favorable to athletic support and performance. Although this may be true for young persons, older individuals often do worse with such shoes because the thicker soles catch more easily on the floor. If the person is used to thinner soles, the foot ordinarily does not make contact with the floor until a lower level is reached compared to thicker soles that contact the floor when the foot is still higher above the floor. It is as though the person wearing thicker soles for the first time is suddenly wearing "extenders" on the bottoms of the feet (the thicker soles) that drag more easily on the floor. Similarly, other shoe characteristics often regarded as beneficial for sports, hiking, or other activities requiring more support may not be good for a person who hopes to have fewer falls. For example, heavier shoes may add weight to the feet that the patient is unaccustomed to. Even the commonly given recommendation banning women's heels is often the wrong advice in persons who may need a slight forward tilt to prevent common backward falls. So let us start with some fresh thinking about what characteristics are desirable and effective in preventive falls.

Some desirable characteristics of shoes that maximize balance and prevent falls are shown in Table 6–5.

Shoes the patient is accustomed to. Wearing shoes the patient is accustomed to, especially in an older person, is an important recommendation because an older person has a more difficult time adapting to a new set of "feet." Shoes are, in a sense, an extension of the feet, the part of the foot that contacts the floor. Any major change in the shoe's outside shape, particularly the sole's shape, thickness, or slope (height of heel) will affect the "feel" of the shoe

Table 6–5. Characteristics of Shoes
that Prevent Falls

Shoes the patient is accustomed to
Flexible
Lightweight
Thin soled
Smooth soled
Small heel, if accustomed
Not "sticky" soled

on the floor. Some modern shoes even have soles that are rounded for walking ease or comfort, but such changes in soles provide an unexpected feel to the foot as it contacts the floor. Letting the patient keep the shoes he is used to, even if not ideal, will be a better choice than changing the shoe type completely when a person is elderly.

Flexible and lightweight. Shoes should be flexible and lightweight so that the movement of the foot, already somewhat limited in old age, is maximized. There are exceptions to this rule (see below) in which there are cases, such as in certain types of severe neuropathy, when it is good to not allow much flexibility at the ankle so that the foot can act as a "unit."

Thin and smooth soles. As discussed at the beginning of this section, thin soles are usually best because they provide the person a better "feel" of the floor. Thicker soles catch more easily on the floor, because if the patient is not used to thick soles, the floor seems to be higher than usual catching the patient unaware. Therefore "athletic shoes," having thicker soles, are not recommended unless the person is used to wearing them much of the time. Smooth soles also have an advantage that seems counterintuitive. It would seem that smooth soles would slip more easily and that shoes with more traction would "grab" the floor better. This is true, but because older persons often shuffle more as they walk, grabbing the floor only leads to a tendency to catch the foot, which increases falls.

Heels. Heels are usually thought of as dangerous and not recommended for those who tend to fall. Although this is often true, there are frequently situations for which a small heel is preferable and prevents falls. If the patient has a tendency to fall backward, a small heel (1–2 inches) can help to keep the patient tilted slightly forward. During the falls examination, we frequently encounter patients (usually women) who purposely wear a small heel because they find that this gives them better balance. This may also apply to men, who may find that wearing a boot with a heel, such as a cowboy boot, may provide better balance for the same reason.

Exceptions. Many exceptions apply to the above guidelines. By analyzing the person's gait and particular disorder, it can be ascertained what type of footwear may be best. Particular attention should be paid to the ankle to ascertain whether it has too little or too much flexibility. Too little flexibility may occur in arthritis, whereas too much flexibility may exist in severe neuropathy in which the foot can no longer be controlled. One recent interesting case illustrates this latter example.

Case illustration. The patient presented with severe neuropathy of the lower legs and feet. This manifested both sensory and motor deficits such that the patient had neither adequate sensation in the feet to feel the floor easily, nor adequate ability to control fine movements of the feet. In particular, the patient could not flex the ankle muscles, resulting in an inability to pull back either the foot as a whole or the toes themselves. This resulted in too much flexibility of the ankle. However, the patient was able to elevate the heel easily while keeping the toes on the floor. For example, when attempting to push a foot switch, as when testing reaction times, the patient could not do so with his toes or front of the foot, but was able to push the switch quickly with the heel while keeping the toes on the ground. From this, it seemed logical that the patient could walk better using the foot as a whole, such as would be more the case while wearing a boot, but had less success when barefoot because the flopping toes and front of the feet tended to drag and get in the way. In this case high boots that would allow the foot to act as a single unit were recommended.

Previous Studies on Falls Prevention

The "Guidelines for the Prevention of Falls in Older Persons," a joint document by the American Geriatrics Society, British Geriatrics Society, and American Academy of Orthopaedic Surgeons Panel on Falls Prevention (2001), evaluated most reputable previous studies up to that time dealing with falls interventions. Analyzing these studies, the authors came up with specific recommendations for various settings (summarized in the section to follow). One interesting finding was that, although many older individuals forget the number of falls they have had, all aging patients should still be screened for falls during routine physical examinations. The screening these authors recommend consists of asking the patient once per year whether there have been any falls. If the answer is "yes" but only one, the person should be evaluated with the "Get Up and Go Test" (see Chapter 5). If this is normal, there need be no further evaluation. If the patient has had multiple falls or is being seen for a visit because of a fall, or demonstrates abnormal gait and/or balance, a fall evaluation should be performed (see Chapter 5).

What Interventions Work?

The AGS (American Geriatrics Society) "*Guidelines*" referenced above recommends various interventions for outpatients as well as inpatients living under various circumstances (see also Chapter 7 for other specific recommendations for inpatients). The AGS recommendations, which were based on available evidence from the several studies reviewed by the authors, are summarized below:

Multifactorial Interventions

For those living in their own homes, multifactorial interventions should include:

Gait training and advice on the use of assistive devices

Review and modification of medicines (especially psychotropics)

Exercise program that contains balance training

Treatment for postural hypotension

Environmental modifications if hazards are present

Treatment of cardiovascular problems including arrhythmia.

For residents in long-term care and assisted living facilities:

Staff education

Gait training and instruction on use of assistive devices

Address medications as above.

For acute hospital settings:

Sufficient evidence is not available to recommend for or against multifactorial interventions.

Single Interventions

Exercise:

Although proven to benefit in preventing falls, the optimal type, duration, or intensity is unclear

Older persons with recurrent falls should have long exercise and balance training that is long-term

Tai Chi is showing promise according to studies, but requires more evaluation to be recommended as the preferred type of exercise.

Environmental modification:

A home assessment should be considered for those at risk for falls who are discharged from the hospital.

Medications:

For patients who have fallen, medications should be reviewed and altered or stopped, as appropriate, with particular attention being given to older patients who take four or more medications or psychotropic medications.

Assistive devices:

> There is no direct evidence that assistive devices used
> alone are of benefit in preventing falls. (Cannot be
> recommended at this time without attention to other
> risk factors; however, they have been included as a part
> of multifactorial interventions that have proven effective.)

Behavioral and educational programs:

> Used in isolation, behavioral and educational programs
> do not reduce falls (should not be done in isolation).

Committee comments on other interventions:

> Hormone replacement therapy, calcium, Vitamin D, or
> antiresorptive agents reduce fracture rates but do not
> reduce the numbers of falls.

> Pacemakers may reduce falls in certain patients (see
> *Guidelines*) but cannot be recommended at this time.

> Specific footwear is not recommended due to lack of
> data.

> Restraints have serious drawbacks that can contribute
> to serious injuries. There is no evidence that they
> reduce falls.

Preventing Injury

Injury from falls in elderly persons is likely because of several factors. Persons in this age group are slower to respond and therefore less able to prevent injury by arresting the fall before it occurs. General body weakness and frailty are common as well as osteoporosis, which can add to the risk of broken bones. If a person is on a blood thinner, this adds to the risk of internal injury after falls. Studies show, however, that risk of falling is not an adequate reason to limit the use of blood thinners in patients for whom these medications are necessary.

Preventing injury consists of modifying the environment and/ or having the patient wear some type of padding such as a hip protector. The environment should be modified so that there are no sharp or dangerous objects to fall onto. Many patients present to our clinic with cuts and other abrasions on their faces, hands, arms, or legs which result from falling onto some low lying or sharp object such as a wooden or glass coffee table. Having more furniture, however, if closely spaced, can give the person something to hold onto or fall up against should a fall occur. Such furniture should be waist high or greater so that the patient does not trip over the furniture. All furniture should be stable so that it does not tip over when fallen against. Although carpeting has been shown to prevent injury, carpeting that is too thick can make a person more likely to fall in the first place because it makes the ground unstable, which renders the "leg" balance system less effective. Carpeting of normal thickness, however, prevents injury because it has been shown that more injuries occur when hitting a hard surfaced floor. Of course area rugs or throw rugs have been shown to be very dangerous because they can be easily tripped over.

Hip Protectors

Hip protectors are not a very popular wardrobe accessory for most people; however, studies have shown that these devices do help prevent injury. In a study reported in the *New England Journal of Medicine*, 1,801 frail elderly adults were assigned either to a group who wore external hip protectors or did not. Among the group wearing the device, only 13 subjects obtained a hip fracture compared to 67 hip fractures in the group not wearing the device (Kannus, Parkkari, Niemi, et al., 2000). Some studies, however, contradict this finding.

When considering what factors help to prevent injury from falls, it is good to remember the concepts presented in Chapter 3 dealing with the physical characteristics needed in the individual who could prevent or stop a fall. These were listed as the attributes of **"strength,"** **"quickness,"** and **"coordination,"** which emphasize the need for exercise. Exercise promotes these attributes; therefore, increasing a patient's strength, quickness, and coordination will help to prevent falls, as well as increase the patient's ability to arrest the fall before it becomes too severe. In this case, we must emphasize the need for "safe" exercise, because it has been found that falls actually increase in many older individuals who start an exercise program. Safe exercise means exercising while holding onto something. This could be a shopping cart, walker, or handrail. Possibly, a person who is frail could exercise while walking and holding onto a partner if the partner is considerably more stable than the potential faller. The use of a walker often has the benefit of helping the person take many more steps per day than if no walker were being used, thereby increasing exercise and the potential for improved balance and strength.

Summary

In summary, the practical prevention strategies presented in this chapter focus on behavior modification in combination with determining the main medical cause leading to falls. It is believed that most falls can be prevented regardless of medical cause with the right application of the behavior modification techniques described. Despite the lack of evidence for walking aids always helping to prevent injury, common sense indicates that the use of these devices do indeed prevent many falls and injuries. One key consideration when recommending such devices is the advice of professionals when choosing the appropriate walking aid so that the device can be suited to the individual needs of the patient.

References

American Geriatrics Society, British Geriatrics Society, and American Academy of Orthopaedic Surgeons Panel on Falls Prevention. (2001). Guidelines for the prevention of falls in older persons. *Journal of the American Geriatric Society, 49,* 664–672.

Aubert, R. E., Herman, W. H., Waters, J., Moore, W., Sutton, D., Peterson, B. L., Bailey, C. M., Koplan, J. P.(1998). Nurse case management to improve glycemic control in diabetic patients in a health maintenance organization: A randomized controlled trial. *Annals of Internal Medicine, 129,* 605–612.

Bandura, A. (1986). *Social foundation of thoughts and action: A social cognitive theory.* Englewood Cliffs, NJ: Prentice-Hall.

Department of Health and Human Services Public Health Service, Office of Disease Prevention and Health Promotion. (1994). *Put prevention into practice* [education and action kit]. Washington, DC: Government Printing Office.

DiMatteo, M. R. (1991). *The psychology of health, illness and medical care: An individual perspective.* Pacific Grove, CA: Brooks/Cole.

Gottman, J. M., & Levenson, R. W. (1999). What predicts change in marital interaction over time? A study of alternative models. *Family Process, 38*(2), 143-158.

Kannus, P., Parkkari, J., Niemi, S., Pasanen, M., Palvanen, M., Jarvinen, M., et al. (2000). Prevention of hip fracture in elderly people with use of a hip protector. *New England Journal of Medicine, 343*(23), 1506-1513.

Kirkhart, R., & Kirkhart, E. (1972). The bruised self: Mending in the early years. In K. Yamamoto (Ed.), *The child and his image: Self concept in the early years.* New York: Houghton Mifflin Company.

Miller, W. R., & Rollnick, S. (1991). *Motivational interviewing: Preparing people to change addictive behavior.* New York: The Guilford Press.

Schwazzer, R. (1992). Self efficacy, physical symptoms and rehabilitation of chronic disease. In R. Schwazzer (Ed.), *Self-efficacy: Thought control of action.* Washington, DC: Hemisphere.

Vogt, H. B., & Kapp, C. (1987). Patient education in primary care practice. *Postgraduate Medicine, 81,* 273-278.

Woolf, S. H., Jonas, S., & Lawrence, R. S. (Eds.). (1995). *Health promotion and disease prevention in clinical practice.* Baltimore: Williams & Wilkins.

CHAPTER 7

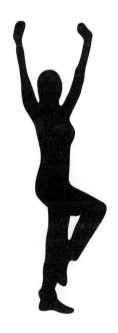

Falls Prevention in Hospitals and Nursing Facilities

Falling among patients in nursing homes or hospitals is a significant problem with about half of nursing home residents in the United States falling at least once per year and approximately 10% of residents incurring serious injuries from these falls (Rubenstein et al., 1988; Rubenstein, Josephson, & Robbins, 1994; Tinetti, 1987). Risk for women who live in nursing homes is approximately 10 times higher for sustaining a hip fracture than if they were living in the community (Scott, Donaldson, & Gallagher, 2003). Among hospitalized patients, falls are one of the most commonly reported incidents (Sutton, Standan, & Wallace, 1994). One paper reports the incidence of falls in hospitals being 0.6 to 2.9 falls annually per bed (Rubenstein et al., 1988). Probably not all falls are reported or even known to the staff.

Many intervention strategies for falls prevention have been tried in hospitals and institutions. Although data on the success of such strategies are limited, one study places reduction of falls in nursing homes at approximately 19% (Ray et al., 1997), and for hospitals, overall reduction of falls by such programs is estimated to be approximately 25% (Oliver, Hopper, & Seed, 2000). These figures indicate that there is still work to be done in reducing falls in hospitals and institutions. Perhaps greater success has not been achieved because most prevention strategies employ a "one size fits all" approach; that is, the same strategy is employed on all patients even though the reasons for falling differ greatly among individuals. Evidence is growing that individualized multifactorial strategies are the most effective (RAND-CMS: U.S. Dept. of Health and Human Services, 2002; Scott, Donaldson, & Gallagher, 2003). The Henry Ford Falls Screening protocol described below is one of the first identification protocols to take a comprehensive individualized approach. This approach evaluates all body systems capable of causing falls, and tailors the prevention strategies to the individual. Using this approach, an **Individualized Falls Prevention Plan** is devised for each patient based on their individual needs.

Falls prevention programs in hospitals or nursing facilities serve several purposes. Patient safety has a major impact on the quality of care patients receive. In addition, various government or regulatory mandates help to motivate falls prevention measures. In addition, institutions may benefit by spotlighting falls prevention programs in their advertising, thus helping to establish their institution as "one of the safest."

Falls prevention programs for institutions should have the following components (Figure 7–1):

1. **Identification.** Screen all patients for falls risk using a broad-based assessment such as the **Henry Ford Falls Screening Protocol** as described. This involves identifying "Target" individuals who either have likelihood of falling or have likelihood of serious injury should they fall. For example,

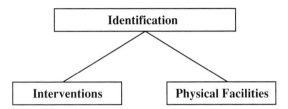

Figure 7–1. Components of an inpatient falls safety program.

patients taking Coumadin have a higher risk of bleeding internally after a fall.

2. **Interventions (prevention programs).** Institute an **Individualized Falls Prevention Plan** for the **"target"** individuals identified. This should include an educational component for staff, patients, and their families or caretakers.

3. **Physical facilities.** Ensure that operating procedures and physical characteristics of the facility are conducive to falls safety for all patients and staff. Safety features such as handrails, grab bars, and others are installed.

Identification

Screening the Fall-Prone Inpatient

A major problem with most existing falls screening measures is that they do not consider enough falls issues. Unlike other disorders, falling can be caused by a multitude of problems; therefore, screening for falls using a small number of criteria is likely to miss many potential fallers. Another problem in screening for potential fallers is that direct observation of the patient is an important aspect left out of many screening measures. By observing the patient, it often is obvious who is at high risk for falls even though they may not possess any of the most common risk factors. For example, a patient may not possess any of the common risk factors such as previous falls or weakness in the legs, but if the patient has a new medical disorder such as postural hypotension, it often is obvious to even a casual observer that the person is at significant risk for falls.

For these reasons, we advocate a more thorough "screening" that should include direct examination of the patient as well as observation of the patient's performance during common activities involving ambulation. We prefer the concept of a "falls screening examination" over a simple questionnaire or quick screening measure that considers only a few criteria. In the "Alvord Falls Screening Examination," based on studies and experiences with the patients referred to the Falls Prevention Clinic at Henry Ford Hospital, a more broad-based approach is taken.

Alvord Falls Screening Examination

The Alvord Falls Screening Examination, which can be used for either inpatients or outpatients is based on elements of the comprehensive Henry Ford Hospital Falls Prevention Clinic's falls assessment (see Chapter 5). The components of that examination were chosen by considering all body systems capable of causing falls, reviewing the scientific literature dealing with "risk factors," as well as considering other previous and current protocols. Evidence of the effectiveness of the comprehensive Henry Ford Falls Prevention Clinic protocol is based on results of an outcomes measure study performed recently on patients attending the clinic (Alvord, Benninger, & Stach, in press). Results showed that 64.7% of the patients attending the clinic decreased the number of falls during the 6-month period following the visits when compared with the number of falls in the 6-month period prior to their visits. Of 22 patients considered "frequent fallers" (those with three or more falls), 59% had not had any falls in the 6-month period following their clinic appointments.

Using this comprehensive approach, remediation measures could then be based directly on the abnormalities found in the assessment. For example, when it was discovered that lower extremity weakness was the main reason for falls, remediation consisted of physical therapy directed at strengthening exercises.

In contrast to the more comprehensive assessment, usually requiring 2 hours, the Alvord Falls Screening Examination consists of assessment of those characteristics found most often among patients attending the comprehensive falls clinic. The goal was to devise a screening protocol that would identify those most at risk, which could be used by those dealing with inpatients or others needing to be screened for which a shorter testing period would be required.

Rationale

When asking patients attending the Falls Prevention Clinic about the circumstances surrounding their falls, it was obvious that both medical and nonmedical factors were involved. The most common medical causes we encountered were **vestibular (inner ear)**, and those involving the **lower extremities (legs and feet)**. Less common but still significant medical causes were **cardiovascular (primarily blood pressure issues)** and **neurological (primarily major disorders such as stroke and degenerative diseases)**. It is recognized, however, that some of the "less common" causes would be quite common among certain patient populations.

As previously mentioned, various "nonmedical" issues were also found to be major causes of falls in our patients. The most common of these were **behavioral (including psychological issues as well as personality factors such as "rushing")**. Less common but still significant nonmedical factors were **"environmental" (lacking safety features in the home)**. Environment is not assessed directly, but is considered an important factor to address in the **remediation component** of the Falls Clinic.

In scoring the examination, failure on any one of the examination areas identifies a person as being at "significant immediate falls risk." We consider it unwise to "grade" risk of falling in terms of "mild," "moderate," or "severe" risk. We also feel that it is unwise to label someone who passes the screening as "not at significant risk of falls." Rather, we simply identify and target individuals who are at significant risk of falling. For persons who pass, we still feel that it is wise to give counseling on falls safety measures along with a handout outlining safety tips and "danger signs" in terms of a person's future health.

Although many risk factors did not "make the cut" and become part of our screening protocol, a common sense approach is still employed in that the tester should have a broad knowledge of other risk factors. This allows the tester to still fail a patient if, for example, there is obvious generalized weakness or other medical issues that would cause the examiner to identify the patient as having an obvious "significant immediate falls risk." Such risk factors, including the use of sedating medications or other factors discussed in Chapter 3 are usually either readily observable or can be noted by a chart review.

Alvord Falls Screening Examination Protocol

The Alvord Falls Screening Examination Protocol is shown in Figure 7–2. Failure in any area constitutes a "fail," signifying significant falls risk. A worksheet is found in Appendix D.

As seen in Figure 7–2, there are several criteria that require a somewhat subjective judgment by the examiner. This approach is probably justifiable, however, because of the complexity of the problem of falling. It is also suggested that those performing the screening receive training and have experience with dizziness and falls evaluations.

		Yes	No
Patient name:			
Dob:			
Date:			
History:	Previous falls? (2 or more in one year, or 1 if injury)	☐	☐
	Medications that are affecting patient's performance? (subjective rating by examiner)	☐	☐
	Room spins?	☐	☐
	Knees give out causing falls?	☐	☐
Vestibular:	Nearly falls when walking while turning head?	☐	☐
	Falls soon when standing on thick foam, with eyes open or closed?	☐	☐
	Abnormal Dix-Hallpike test?	☐	☐

Figure 7–2. Alvord Falls Screening. *continues*

		Yes	No
Lower extremities:	Reduced strength or feeling	☐	☐
	Significant pain or weakness when walking?	☐	☐
Psych/Behavioral:	Dementia?	☐	☐
	Depression?	☐	☐
	Risky habits (rushing, carrying on stairs, etc.)?	☐	☐
Cardiovascular:	Orthostatic hypotension?	☐	☐
	Irregular pulse or palpitations or other heart disease that cause symptoms?	☐	☐
Neurologic:	Stroke, Parkinson's, or other neurologic disorder that affects movements?	☐	☐
Informal balance:	"Up and Go test" abnormal (nearly falls or >20 seconds)	☐	☐
	Unsteady gait?	☐	☐
	Tinetti abnormal—unsteady when turns in circle in place, when nudged, turning in place, reaching high, picking up, using stairs?	☐	☐
	Functional reach—falls reaching less than 12 inches?	☐	☐
Vision:	Vision corrected is 20/50 or worse binocular	☐	☐
Other:	Other obvious risk factor?		

Pass/Fail:

Comments:

Figure 7–2. *continued*

Controversial Aspects of Screening

The subject of screening has some controversial aspects. For example, there are those who feel that only performing a screening is
not enough because inherent in any screening is the possibility of
missing a disorder that might be picked up in a more complete
evaluation. Therefore, some would argue against screening on the
grounds that everyone should have as complete evaluation as possible. On the other hand, advocates of screening argue that it is
unlikely that a complete evaluation will take place for many individuals; therefore, screening will at least pick up those who would
otherwise not be tested at all. It is, therefore, worthwhile discussing
the possible rationale for doing large-scale screenings. Prior authors
have pointed out that screening large numbers of individuals for a
disorder is not always wise depending on a "cost–benefit" analysis.
Some of the key issues to consider when deciding the efficacy
of screening for a particular disorder (Frankenburg, 1975; North,
1976; Northern & Downs, 1991) are discussed below.

Occurrence Frequent Enough or Consequences Serious Enough to Warrant Mass Screening

This condition appears to be easily met considering the high prevalence of fallers and the dire potential consequences involved in
falling as outlined in Chapter 1.

Amenability to Treatment of Prevention That Will Forestall or Change the Expected Outcome

It is clearly evident from the literature cited in Chapter 1 that many
falls are preventable to a significant extent.

Availability of Facilities for Diagnosis and Treatment

There are probably not enough current clinics for the purpose of
assessing and preventing falls. On the positive side, adequate numbers of trained professionals from several disciplines potentially are
available to perform these assessments and prevention interventions. Falls clinics are becoming more common but still are lacking
in many geographic areas.

Cost of Screening Reasonably Commensurate with Benefits to the Individual

The screening test proposed here has low relative cost and the benefits to the individual are high considering the extreme consequences to the frail elderly who fall as well as to the institutions that house them (see Chapter 1).

In summary, it is apparent from the above analysis that the benefits versus costs are favorable for screening for falls, particularly for inpatients and possibly for outpatients who have had close calls or previous falls but cannot undergo the comprehensive evaluation.

Assessment Measures by Other Investigators

Risk Factors for Inpatients

Risk factors for hospitalized inpatients differ from those of outpatients because inpatients are acutely ill and not in their familiar environment. On the other hand, they are not performing their daily routine activities, which may put them at risk in other ways. Being an inpatient may either increase or decrease one's risk of falls. In a review by Oliver et al. (2004), the following risk factors for inpatients emerged consistently:

- gait instability
- agitated confusion
- urinary incontinence/frequency
- falls history
- certain medications (especially sedative/hypnotics).

In an interesting article, Eagle et al. (1999) compared three different methods or scales for predicting falls of inpatients which included some scored screening measures for predicting those most likely to fall. The conclusion was that the formal instruments were time consuming and in some cases no better than the nurses' judgment. In our judgment, formal instruments do have the advantage of being consistent and offer a means of comparison between patients or when the same patient is tested more than once.

Scored Falls Risk Assessment Tests

Scored falls risk assessment tests allow documentation of a patient's numerical score concerning various risk factors, personal performance, or patient circumstances. One advantage of scored screening measures is that they are quickly administered. A possible disadvantage is that each covers a limited number of factors rather than being a system based or more comprehensive evaluation. Certain patients who do not have the risk factors covered by a particular screening measure could be expected to "fall through the cracks" (no pun intended). Nevertheless, scored scales can be expected to identify most patients at risk for falls.

Morse Fall Scale

The Morse Fall Scale is a very practical scale based largely on the nurse's observations of the patient plus review of past medical records and history (Morse, Morse, & Tylko, 1989). Elements considered indicative of future falls include:

- Patient has more than a single diagnosis
- Use of an ambulatory aid or the patient "clutches" for support
- Patient is attached to an intravenous apparatus or heparin lock
- Gait is stooped, uses short steps or shuffling gait
- Difficulty rising to walk or needs assistance
- Patient's answer to the question, "Can you go to the bathroom alone, or are you permitted up?" differs from what is indicated in the ambulatory orders (this response is used as an informal assessment of mental status).

Points are assigned according to the above criteria. A strong point of this scale is that it includes factors that are based on direct observation of the patient relating to patient abilities.

Hendrich II

Somewhat similar to the Morse scale, the Hendrich II (Hendrich, Bender, & Nyhuis, 2003) assigns points based on various risk factors:

■ Confusion/disorientation
■ Depression
■ Altered elimination
■ Dizziness/vertigo
■ Gender (male)
■ Administration of prescribed antiepileptics or benzodiazepines
■ Performance on the "Get-up-and-go" test.

A strong point of the Hendrich II is that it includes the specific medical conditions of dizziness or vertigo while also considering the patient's practical performance (Get-up-and-go test).

Berg Functional Mobility Test

The Berg balance test, formally called Berg Functional Mobility Test, is a widely used test of practical functional balance and mobility that assesses such items as ability to sit and stand unsupported for a particular amount of time, reach forward, retrieve an object from the floor, turn to look behind, and others. Each ability is rated on a 4-point scale ranging from "unable [to do] without help" to fully able to perform the task without supervision. This scale allows the facility to document improvement of the patient over time. The test has been studied to determine its sensitivity for predicting falls. An article by Bogle Thorbahn and Newton (1996) discusses factors that affect the sensitivity of the Berg test.

STRATIFY

The STRATIFY falls assessment tool was developed in the United Kingdom for use with hospital inpatients (Oliver et al., 1998). Patients are scored on six items, namely, previous falls; mental status is confused, disoriented, or agitated; abnormal vision; alterations in urination; difficulty with transfers; and decreased mobility. Authors claim good sensitivity and specificity, high predictive validity, and reproducibility. The items are reportedly easy to assess and the tester does not require extensive training.

Other Falls Screening Tests

It is likely that using only the tests above will miss many potential fallers. Shorter screening tests, which are even less extensive, are bound to miss many of the important factors known to cause falls. Nevertheless, screening is sometimes all that is allowable in a particular setting. For more information on shorter screening measures, the reader is referred to a study by Thomas and Lane (2005), which retrospectively assessed four falls screening measures, the Up and Go test, Functional Reach Test, one-leg stance test (OLST), and balance subsection of the Performance Oriented Mobility Assessment (B-POMA). Their findings were that the OLST and B-POMA have potential as screening tools but that confirmation in a prospective study would be necessary.

Summary of Screening Measures

As stated previously, it is likely that "falls screening" requires consideration of multiple body systems as well as direct examination of the patient. Some of the tools described above either contain too few criteria or do not require direct examination of the patient's abilities.

Interventions

Many strategies have been employed for many years to reduce falls in hospitals and nursing homes due to the high incidence of such falls. Although hospitals differ from nursing homes in many respects, most studies to date have dealt with nursing homes in terms of studying effectiveness of these various strategies. In a comprehensive review of such studies, Scott, Donaldson, and Gallagher (2003) analyzed the reported effectiveness of the various strategies employed to date. In summing up their study, the authors state that the evidence is growing that individualized multifactorial strategies are the most effective but that some of the commonly used methods have not yet been proven effective. For example, although assistive devices no doubt benefit many individuals, there is no strong research evidence to back this up. The same thing holds for isolated medication reviews and organizational changes, although it is logical that these measures would be of benefit. On the other hand, there is strong evidence for the effectiveness of environmental modifications and certain types of exercise.

What Works?

Literature reviewers bemoan the fact that few well-designed controlled studies are available that show the effectiveness of the various strategies for hospital use.

Strategies Still Under Study

Below are short summaries of research findings to date on the various strategies listed; however, it is likely that many of these are useful and that future studies will prove their benefit.

> **Bed alarms:** Studies disagree, with some studies showing limited benefit. This could be due to the fact that too many alarms are used for various reasons in hospitals and are sometimes ignored.
>
> **Identification bracelets:** Evidence of the usefulness of bracelets or other means of identifying potential fallers is lacking at present. This measure is still looked on favorably because it incurs very little cost. It is at least a visible sign to relatives and others that the institution is doing something to prevent falls.
>
> **Bed rails:** There is little doubt that bed rails sometimes keep persons with certain disorders from falling out of bed; however, many patients fall from bed despite the use of bed rails. In some cases, patients have fallen farther because they have climbed over bed rails before falling. In contrast, having the bed lower to the floor and closer to the bathroom seems to definitely help.
>
> **Restraints:** Restraints of various forms for bed or wheelchair are a controversial measure and of

questionable benefit for falls prevention. Many patients have fallen despite the restraint or have injured themselves because of it. On the other hand, using latex mesh on chairs prevents slipping. Studies are still needed in this area.

Interventions Already Shown to Be Helpful

Individualized falls assessment: Each patient's individual capabilities and risk factors should be assessed rather than applying a "one size fits all" philosophy to falls prevention. Use a **Personalized Falls Prevention Plan** consisting of strategies tailored to the individual based on finding from the broad-based falls screening described above (Henry Ford Falls Screening protocol). In most cases, the patient's own medical condition relating to falls in conjunction with the observed capabilities for balance and mobility noted on the screening will dictate what prevention measures need to be employed.

Location of bed: Placing the patient's bed close to the bathroom.

Assistance when walking: Help with toileting in individuals who have had a change or increase in toileting requirements.

Transfer assistance: Assisting appropriate patients with transfers has been shown to help to prevent falls.

Proximity of personal items and call button: Having necessary personal items close to the bed as well as an easy to reach call button are beneficial.

Chair close to bed: Having a stable chair close to the bed gives the patient something to hold onto when attempting to walk as well as something to fall back into should a fall occur.

Adequate lighting available: Having the light switch by the bed or the light on in the bathroom with the door partially open have been shown to prevent falls.

Foam bedside pads: Foam bedside pads for a person to fall out of bed onto have been found to prevent injury for those falling out of bed; however, these can actually increase falls because a person cannot sense the floor as well with the feet. The latter is especially true when a person has any degree of vestibular dysfunction as do a high percentage of aging individuals. Foam bedside pads should probably only be used when a person falls out of bed. Although many persons fall when first getting out of bed, having something to hold onto, such as a stable chair by the side of the bed, is a better idea for most individuals.

Physical Facilities

Although institutions providing health care generally have features that are conducive to falls prevention such as **grab bars** in bathrooms, **handrails** in hallways, and **nonslip floors**, other environmental changes would improve the falls situation.

The following checklist should be used for a **fall-proof** environment:

Spills? Spills frequently occur in hospitals in and around patient areas. Floors having certain multicolored surfaces make spills more difficult to notice. Mark or clean up all spills immediately. Spills having materials that may cause health risks such as contaminated fluids should be marked until proper cleanup procedures can be carried out.

Distances too far? Having something substantial to hold onto such as a chair closed by the bed is one of the most effective means of preventing falls. In contrast, large open areas in which the patient has to navigate without anything to hold onto can be trouble. Having something to hold onto between the patient's bed and the bathroom is important. Placing the bed closer to the bathroom is a possible way to solve the problem. Having more furniture, waist high or higher, is a good idea. Furniture gives the person something to hold onto as well as something to fall up against instead of the floor.

Light too low? Adequate lighting is crucial to good balance for most fall-prone individuals. Because these patients usually have some type of impaired balance, they need their vision to be maximally functioning to more effectively compensate for their lack of balance. Environments having low light greatly increase the risk of falls. Having a lights witch close to the bed is an ideal way to accomplish the goal of having adequate light when it is needed.

Bed too high? Because many patients fall from their beds (see discussion above on restraints) having the bed as low as possible helps to minimize injury from falls. Hospital beds are typically high to aid the nurse or doctor when performing a procedure. Many beds can be lowered, however. Beds having wheels should be locked at all times

Level of rounding too low? As much as administrators hate to hear it, patients who fall frequently need a higher level of supervision than average patients. If left alone long enough, such patients always seem to find a way to fall, no matter how many safety measures have been adopted. Such patients will only be safe when walking with someone or being assisted with transfers. More frequent rounding to check on frequently falling patients is necessary to prevent falls.

Safety features installed? Standard safety features for bathrooms, hallways, and other open areas should be installed. These include **nonslip surfaces** in showers or tubs, **grab bars** in appropriate areas, and **hand rails** in hallways and on steps or ramps. **Half rails on beds**, **alarms**, and **bedside pads** are appropriate only for certain types of fallers (see above discussion).

Summary

Falls are numerous in institutions and hospitals. Being in a new unfamiliar environment as well as being ill adds to the already high risk of falls for the aging or sick patient. The three components of a falls prevention program include **identification**, implementation of **interventions**, and modification of the **environment** for falls safety.

References

Alvord, L., Benninger, M., & Stach, B. (in press). An otolaryngology based Multidisciplinary falls clinic. *Ear, Nose and Throat Journal.*

Bogle Thorbahn, L. D., & Newton, R. A. (1996). Use of the Berg Balance Test to predict falls in elderly persons. *Physical Therapy, 76*(6), 576-583.

Eagle, D. J., Salama, S., Whitman, D., Evans, L. A., Ho, E., & Olde, J. (1999). Comparison of three instruments in predicting accidental falls in selected inpatients in a general teaching hospital. *Journal of Gerontology Nursing, 25*(7), 40-45.

Frankenburg, W. K., & Camp, B. W. (1975). *Pediatric screening tests.* Springfield, IL: Charles C Thomas.

Hendrich, A. L., Bender, P. S., & Nyhuis, A. (2003). Validation of the Hendrich II falls risk model: A large concurrent case/control study of hospitalized patients. *Applied Nursing Research, 16*(1), 9-21.

McCollam, M. E. (1995). Evaluation and implementation of a research-based falls assessment innovation. *Nursing Clinics of North America, 30*(3), 507-514.

McFarlane-Kolb, H. (2004). Falls risk assessment, multitargeted interventions and the impact on hospital falls. *International Journal of Nursing Practice, 10*(5), 199.

Morse, J. M., Morse, R. M., & Tylko, S. J. (1989). Development of a scale to identify the fall-prone patient. *Canadian Journal on Aging, 8*(4), 366-367.

North, F. A. (1975). In W. K. Frankenburg & B. W. Camp (Eds.), *Pediatric screening tests* (chap 4). Springfield IL: Charles C. Thomas.

Northern, J. L., & Downs, M. P. (1991). Screening for hearing disorders. In J. L. Northern & M. P. Downs (Eds.), *Hearing in children* (4th ed.). Baltimore: Williams & Wilkins.

Oliver, D., Britton, M., Seed, P., Martin, F. C., & Hopper, A. H. (1998). A 6-point risk score predicted which elderly patients would fall in hospital. *British Medical Journal, 315*,1049–1053.

Oliver, D., Daly, F., Martin, F., & McMurdo, M. E. T. (2004). Risk factors and risk assessment tools for falls in hospital in-patients: A systematic review. *Age and Ageing, 33*, 122–130.

RAND-CMS. (2002). *Healthy Aging Project. Draft evidence report and evidence-based recommendation: Falls prevention interventions in the Medicare population.* Washington, DC: U.S. Department of Health and Human Services Centers for Medicare and Medicaid Services.

Ray, W. A., Taylor, J. A., Meador, K. G., Thapa, P. B., Brown, A. K., Kajihara, H. K., et al. (1997). A randomized trial of consultation service to reduce falls in nursing homes. *Journal of the American Medical Association, 278*(7), 557–562.

Rubenstein L. Z., Josephson, K. R., & Robbins, A. S. (1994). Falls in the nursing home. *Annals of Internal Medicine, 121*, 442–451.

Rubenstein, L. Z., Robbins, A. S., Schulman, B. L., Rosado, J., Osterweil, D., & Josephson, K. R. (1988). Falls and instability in the elderly. *Journal of the American Geriatric Society, 36*, 266–278.

Scott, V. J., Donaldson, M., & Gallagher, E. M. (2003, September). A review of the literature on best practices in falls prevention for residents of long-term care facilities. *Long Term Care Falls Review.*

Sutton, J., Standan, P., & Wallace, A. (1994). Incidence and documentation of patient accidents in hospital. *Nursing Times, 90*, 29–35.

Thomas, J. I., & Lane, J. V. (2005). A pilot study to explore the predictive validity of 4 measures of falls risk in frail elderly patients. *Archives of Physical Medicine and Rehabilitation, 86*(8), 1636–1640.

Tinetti, M. E. (1987). Factors associated with serious injury during falls by ambulatory nursing home residents. *Journal of the American Geriatric Society, 35*, 644–648.

CHAPTER 8

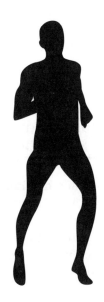

Case Studies

Among other things, the following cases demonstrate these important principles:

1. that much valuable information exists "below the surface" of what the patient initially says,
2. that solutions to falls are often nonmedical and that friends or family can help the patient to arrive at his or her own solutions that are mutually acceptable, and lastly
3. that in some frequent fallers nothing much can be done except to try to prevent injury when the inevitable falls occur.

As outlined in the behavior modification section (see Chapter 6), more recent behavioral modification techniques stress the importance of having the patient come to a realization of the causes of his or her own problem as well as the possible solutions. Case 1 demonstrates the format of the Falls Clinic as described in narrative fashion. Cases 2 through 6 are presented in a typical case-study format.

Case 1: Narrative Description of a "Typical Falls Clinic Visit"

Mary, a 78-year-old, fit but somewhat frail looking female, is sitting in the examination room by herself when I enter. We are in the "Part 2" falls clinic visit, Mary already having attended Part 1, which consisted of typical vestibular testing of VNG, rotational chair, and posturography. I am accompanied today by Dr. Hasbro (name changed) who is an internal medicine resident and we will be joined by the physical therapist toward the end of the visit.

At the first visit, I had taken Mary's history. Besides the typical vestibular questions, Mary had been asked questions specifically regarding her falls. The question "How many falls have you had in the past 6 months?" had produced the response "six" from Mary, meaning that, if she was being honest, she was falling an average of about once per month.

"Tell me about some of your falls," I ask.

"Well, I can be doing just about anything and for no reason I just fall," she responds.

Because that is a vague but all too common answer, I persist in searching for how the falls occur. Answers are all negative to the questions, "Are you tripping?" "Do your knees or legs 'give out'?" or "Do you feel weak before you fall?"

But I finally hit "pay dirt" with the questions, "Are you more likely to fall after you first get up?" and "Are you more off-balance when you turn quickly?" which are both answered with, "Yes, sometimes I guess."

I also note one more telling response, that she "rushes to do everything" and that it is "just my personality, I always rush."

After the history questions have been administered, we next review the results of the first visit's vestibular testing. The conversation went something like this.

"During our last visit, we tested mainly your "inner ear" balance system. Today we will assess your other "balance systems," legs, eyes, and other possible reasons for falling. At the last visit, we did find one "inner ear" abnormality. Did you follow up with the referring ENT?"

"Yes, earlier today, Dr. Jones told me I had "uncompensated 'something,' and that there was nothing he could do about it, but that you would be giving me some exercises."

"That's right. I'll tell you about the exercises or possible physical therapy for the "uncompensated vestibulopathy" at the end of the visit. Did he explain what that means?"

"Yes, something about one ear being damaged for balance, but I didn't get it all."

I next explain a layman's version of uncompensated nonspecific vestibulopathy, which includes a description about the inner ears also having a balance function, and so forth, but I tell her that we will discuss this in more detail at the end of the visit.

Aided by Dr. Hasbro, we next proceed with the Part 2 "Falls Visit" the details of which are given in Chapter 5, but which include "bedside" assessments of all other body systems possibly contributing to falls, including informal balance tests such as the Tenneti tests for gait and balance, tests of lower muscle strength and feeling, blood pressures and pulse while lying compared to standing (orthostatics), vision testing using a standard Snellen chart, as well as assessment of contrast vision, mood and cognition testing, reaction times for hand and foot, and a chart review to assess overall medical conditions and medications. Each of these tests represents a possible "risk factor" for falls.

Next, the physical therapist arrives and performs a screening of the patient's potential benefit from physical therapy. While the physical therapist is doing this, we are going over the chart in another room and beginning to write the report so that it can be presented at the end of the visit during the counseling portion.

The physical therapist now comes to us with her results, stating that Mary has normal strength and feeling and does not need physical therapy for general strength or gait purposes. Dr. Hasbro, from his chart review, has not found any past or present ototoxic medications, but does note that the patient is on three medications to lower blood pressure.

During our discussion, the bottom line assessment by the team is that Mary's "main problem" is her vestibulopathy, with the lesser contributing problems being the drop in blood pressure when standing after sitting for a long time as well as her tendency to "rush." That the vestbulopathy is the "main problem" was ascertained from her descriptions of her falls, that they most often occur when she is turning, and less often after just getting up.

The final portion of the visit consists of a counseling session in which the patient's family and the team members all participate if possible. Mary's daughter had been sitting in the hall and now joins us.

"We would like to go over all the results and offer some suggestions," I say.

It is our policy to stress the positive during these sessions. With some people who are somewhat worse off than Mary, it can be quite discouraging to the patient to be presented with a long list of deficiencies. After all, most persons in their eighties will have several issues that could possibly affect their balance. Rather, we find it more effective to go over the positive points about the patient's balance abilities and then end with the issues needing improvement. It is also helpful to try to arrive at one "main cause" of falls that can be given first priority for remediation. In Mary's case, the main cause could also have been considered her "rushing." Although rushing is a behavioral and not a medical characteristic, sometimes changing behavior is the only workable solution. In Mary's case, however, the vestbulopathy is a correctable condition and so that aspect of her problem was given the greatest attention.

"You certainly have a lot going for you in terms of your balance ability. The physical therapist comments that you are exceptionally strong and have good feeling in your legs and feet. You are not burdened by painful arthritis or other pain that is causing you to walk abnormally. In fact, your gait is normal. You do walk a little quickly. Have you always walked that quickly?"

"Yes that's just me."

"O.K. The best news is that we all feel that your falling can be corrected. This is not just a case of your getting old and having to live with it, as you once commented. The most likely "main problem" causing your falls is the inner ear disorder, the "uncompensated vestibulopathy." That can usually be greatly improved if not completely solved with some rehabilitation. A physical therapist can direct you in this or, if you are disciplined, we can try some self-directed home exercises. The problem is, they make you somewhat dizzier than at first, and so you have to be persistent and disciplined. Also contributing to your falls are your tendency to rush as well as the drop in blood pressure when you get up after sitting for a long time or lying down. Dr. Hasbro would like to speak to you a little bit more about that."

Dr. Hasbro now asks whether she obtained all the blood pressure medicines from the same doctor. It is determined that she had once obtained a "water pill" possibly affecting the blood pressure from a separate doctor. Dr. Hasbro recommends she consult with her primary physician regarding these medications, and this suggestion is also mentioned in our report.

Regarding her rushing habit, we have a rather lengthy discussion about her various daily habits, making suggestions for other slower "habits" that may replace her bad rushing habits. One suggestion is to carry a portable phone that can act both as a safety alarm should she fall when alone in her home as well as a means to avoid rushing to answer the phone.

In addition, we presented the concepts of "SafeWalk," a walking technique we have developed designed to minimize falls risk. The technique involves slower turning methods as well helping the patient to develop other safer habits of moving about.

The physical therapist also offers some specific recommendations regarding home safety issues and gives a handout listing common home hazards. She asks Mary's daughter if she will help her mother add features such as grab bars in the bathroom, a seat for the shower, and other safety items.

Next, the self-directed vestibular rehabilitation exercises are presented. It was felt that, as the daughter is involved in her mother's care, there is high likelihood of her complying with the exercises and that, if she does not, the daughter can report this and we can resort to more consistent vestibular rehabilitation involving a physical therapist.

Finally, we provide the patient with a copy of the final report. This had been finished while the physical therapist was performing her portion of the evaluation. To involve the patient more in the way of accountability, we tell the patient that we will be calling her in a few months and that at that time we hope that she will be able to report no more falls.

Case 2: "Needing to Change Location of Bedroom?"

Principle Demonstrated in This Case

This case demonstrates the importance of the patient and family themselves determining their own best solutions for falls prevention.

The Problem

Audrey (name changed), an agile, strong but extremely thin 79-year-old "faller," lives with her son in his home. She presented to the clinic with her daughter who adds that her problem is a bit worse than Audrey describes it. "I have a little trouble with my balance and fall sometimes, mainly when I get up too quickly, but sometimes just when I'm walking." As is often the case, the patient was downplaying the problem a bit, but the daughter helped to fill in some intriguing details. She had had a toe amputated not too long ago in an attempt to help her gait problem due to "hammer toe," a disorder causing the toe to be pulled backward due to a too tight tendon. The daughter also described her mother as someone who is stubborn and rushes.

On examining the patient's record, recent balance function tests including VNG and rotational chair testing, had shown "normal results for vestibular function." Watching the patient walk, however, she deviated to the left every few steps. On examination of her feet, a probable reason for the deviated gait became apparent. There was a moderately deformed left foot due to a combination of "hammer toe," bunions, and a missing second toe that had been removed a year ago in an attempt to solve the abnormal gait due to the hammer toe. Also of significance, the patient was orthostatic in that her blood pressure dropped 16 systolic points lying to standing, with the pulse increasing 10 points.

On the positive side, the patient also passed the informal balance tests, although because of her rather slight build, she quite easily fell backward with a slight push to the sternum.

Information "Below the Surface"

As is often the case, the information obtained after the formal testing was completed was revealing. When describing her bedroom, Audrey said that she sleeps in a very small room, a kind of combination between a den and a closet, which is right next to the front door. Our conversation had centered on whether or not she could use a bedside commode to solve the need to rush to the bathroom at night, a very dangerous practice. She had said that her bedroom was not large enough to even accommodate a bedside commode. Her daughter confirmed that seeming excuse, telling me that indeed she did sleep in a room next to the front door. When asked why that was the case, Audrey said that she had chosen that room because her son had not been home very much at night when she first started living there. She felt that if she slept near the front door then she would be able to hear an intruder if one should come in. This location of the bedroom made her feel safe. When I inquired whether or not her son were still gone at night, she said "No, lately my son has stopped having to be gone at night" and so she said "I guess I wouldn't have to have my bedroom there anymore." The daughter agreed that this could probably be accomplished. A bedside commode would then be possible.

Audrey had come to this satisfactory conclusion herself, which is a much more likely way of getting the patient to agree to a change. The patient is following through with the blood pressure issue, but one of the main solutions arrived at was a nonmedical family decision that was achieved through counseling. Although medical solutions to the problems of the urinary incontinence and postural hypotension would be ideal, the main goal of the falls clinic is to help arrive at a practical solution that can work immediately. We never know whether the recommended medical solutions will be successful or not and we only have this one opportunity for the patient to attend the falls clinic, so we made the best of it.

Results of Testing

Abnormal Results

Postural hypotension. Blood pressure drops 16 points when standing after lying for 5 minutes.

Rushes to the bathroom at night. She has a urinary problem that requires her to get to the bathroom quickly in order not to soil her bed or clothing.

Abnormal gait. Deviates to the left side every few steps. Walks quickly.

Foot deformities. On the left foot, the second toe has been amputated. She also has other toes having "hammer toe" effect in that the first knuckle of the toe is pulled upward deforming the toe. There are also significant bunions, right foot greater than left.

Normal Results

Balance function tests are essentially normal for vestibular function, although there are a few oculomotor abnormalities. Informal balance testing is also essentially normal (the patient can even stand on thick foam for several seconds with eyes closed without falling); however, the patient is somewhat unstable in that she is easily pushed on the sternum to a backward fall. Strength is good, although a bit reduced in her left hip. Eyesight and contrast vision are normal. The patient does not live alone.

Immediate Solution

Switch bedrooms to accommodate a bedside commode more easily. Wait after standing for 1 minute before walking. Be evaluated by physical therapist for cane or walker. Incorporate other routine safety suggestions.

Medical Solutions

See her primary care provider to address the postural hypotension.

CASE STUDIES 213

What We Learned

This case demonstrates the importance of spending time discussing the living arrangements and personal habits of the patient. If the evaluation had stopped after the testing, the real reasons for rushing to the bathroom would never have surfaced. The patient would have just been given a cane or walker and sent back to her primary care provider without getting to the root of one of the major problems. In this case, the patient's reason for staying in an odd bedroom location made sense to her at the time, but this was eventually determined to be unnecessary now. This self-determined solution will likely be carried out, whereas the medical conditions may or may not be successfully solved.

Case 3: "Legs Too Weak to Support Present Weight"

Principle Demonstrated in This Case

Occasionally a patient will comment that he or she "cannot stand for more than a couple of minutes." This can be due to a variety of problems including neuromuscular, osteoskeletal, or just a general medical condition causing pain or weakness. One of the reasons causing inability to stand for very long is simply being overweight, which is sometimes coupled with weakness in the legs. Falling is, of course, more prevalent in persons who have trouble simply standing. If you add any additional problems to this, which are common in the aging population such as slowed reaction time or neuropathy, then the situation presents an even higher risk for falls. The present case demonstrates a patient with a normal vestibular balance system but who is overweight, has weakened legs, and slower than normal reaction times.

The Problem

Nancy, a 66-year-old female, is a short woman approximately 4½ feet tall but weighing 205 pounds. She speaks mainly Polish but is accompanied by her daughter who translates for her. She says that she has experienced about 20 falls in the past 6 months. She claims that falls occur onto her knees while she is walking when suddenly she cannot move her right leg. Nancy lives alone. Previous to and during a trip to Poland a few months ago, she had presented to the ENT department for dizziness described as a "spinning sensation" that lasts approximately 5 to 10 minutes. The dizzy episodes lasted approximately one-half hour and would usually occur on rising in the morning, although some episodes occurred during the day or night. There is no loss of consciousness." She no longer has the dizziness but continues to fall. Recent vestibular testing was normal.

Results of Testing

Abnormal Results

Left knee and hip are reduced in strength.

Slower than normal reaction times for hand and foot.

Falls or near falls on most informal balance tests, including turning a small circle in place

Abnormal "unsteady" deviating gait.

Normal Results

Normal orthostatics (no drop in blood pressure lying to standing).

Immediate Solution

This patient presents the unusual situation of having frequent falls, but normal vestibular balance sensation (normal vestibular tests). It is most likely that her current falls problem is due to her legs not having adequate strength for her current weight. Particularly her left leg is weak at the knee and hip, due in part to her previous car accident but perhaps more recently to less activity. A second problem is that her reaction speed of the feet is slower than normal, especially on the left side.

Safe exercise, with the consent of her primary doctor, would be beneficial. Safe exercise means always having something to hold onto. A list of home safety features was given to the patient.

Medical Solutions

A complete physical examination with review of medications may also be beneficial.

What We Learned

Adequate legs strength for a particular weight and height is necessary to prevent falls. The patient's "dizziness," which is no longer present although the falls are, is a "red herring" and not the main cause of her dizziness. The comment of not being able to stand for very long is a major clue to the problem. Normal vestibular function further confirms that balance is not her main problem. Barring central nervous system problems, her leg strength to weight and height ratio is the probable cause of her falls.

Case 4

Principle Demonstrated in This Case

Falling is often due to a combination of factors.

The Problem

This 75-year-old female patient has had four or more falls in the past 6 months. Her left knee will sometimes give our when first standing, but she feels that her falls are due to "balance problems." She falls mainly forward or sideward. She reports not being able to stand for very long, but can stand longer when wearing her back brace, which is for degenerative changes in the lumbar spine. She does experience some dizziness described as spinning in the morning or late at night. Current medical issues include arthritis, hypertension, hyperlipidemia, and hypothyroidism.

Information "Below the Surface"

The patient says that she is less active since her husband died a few months ago. This is reason to suspect depression or perhaps she has changed her lifestyle significantly to involve less activity.

Test Results

Abnormal Results

In the patient's lower extremities:

Strength is 3/5 in the left knee, but 4/5 in the hips, right knee, and ankles bilaterally.

Feeling is less in the left foot to light touch than right, but overall, sensation is within normal limits bilaterally.

Gait: Her daughter has observed that sometimes when she is walking, when she turns, her body turns but her feet don't always turn along with her body.

Normal Results

Orthostatics: Normal, no significant change lying 5 minutes to standing.

Informal balance testing: The patient is somewhat unsteady but probably does not have vestibulopathy. Romberg and tandem Romberg are normal; patient can turn a small circle in place in either direction. She is unsteady on foam but can stand for a few seconds with eyes closed. Hallpikes are negative bilaterally.

Immediate Solution

The patient's balance difficulties most likely are leg related, in that her current weight combined with lack of strength in the left knee are probably the biggest factors. Her inability to simply stand for a few minutes is added evidence of this. Her "balance abnormality" is likely not due to a vestibular disorder, although this cannot be positively ruled out without formal testing. Spinning is not a main complaint but is more of an afterthought in her description of her imbalance and falls.

Medical Solutions

Recommendations include in-home physical therapy with the goal of improving gait and balance. She has also agreed to the use of a wheeled walker at least when going from the house to the car, which is the location where she has the most difficulty. We went over several ideas and a list of home safety features, a few of which were lacking.

We asked her to contact us if the symptoms of spinning became significant or more severe, so that we could arrange for formal balance function testing at the main campus ENT department.

What We Learned

Falling can be due to a combination of factors, in this case being overweight and having a weak knee. Not being able to stand for very long is not always due to being overweight. Although the patient was mildly obese, the knee problem is probably the greater cause of her falling.

Case 5

Principle Demonstrated in This Case

Having the patient determine his or her own solution(s) is the most effective way to solve falls problems.

The Problem

The patient, who is a 72-year-old nun, lives alone in a retirement community apartment. She has numerous falls, three in the past month that can occur under any circumstance. She fell in the grocery store for no apparent reason, fell going down some steps, and fell recently in her bathroom when she suddenly felt "off-balance." As a nun, she has the duty to perform prayers during regular religious services in which she must carry a book up to the stand and then read from the book. She feels very off balance when carrying the book.

The most significant past medical problem possibly relating to dizziness is a previous otologic surgery for decompression of an artery affecting the acoustic nerve on the left side. She has no hearing of the left side.

Other medical history includes:

1. Osteoarthritis.
2. Asthma.
3. Mild obesity.
4. History of osteopenia, though most recent bone density was normal.
5. Severe depression.

Information "Below the Surface"

None.

Results of Testing

Abnormal Results

Central nervous system signs were the most significant abnormal finding. These included sudden tremor at times when standing lasting several seconds, inability to perform many of the routine motor tasks during the strength examination including inability to maintain pressure with her foot on the examiner's hand.

Vestibular: Recent VNG, rotational chair, and posturography examination showed bilateral vestibular weakness in conjunction with several central vestibular signs.

Postural hypotension: A drop of systolic blood pressure greater than 20 points lying to standing (lying = 144/79, standing = 111/73).

Informal balance tests: Abnormal gait characterized by constant unsteadiness and near falls.

Lower extremity complaints: Arthritis in the knees with past left knee surgery several years ago, weakness in the left hip.

Normal Results

Normal feeling in lower extremities.

Results Summary

The patient's falling appears most likely to be due to a combination of postural hypotension and a significant central nervous system disorder that is as yet unidentified as to specific diagnosis. She is currently being assessed by a neurologist.

Solutions

Although there may be future medical intervention that will significantly affect this patient's falls situation, we felt it best to make immediate recommendations that could be applied to her current situation. We told her that, although her medical situation may improve due to future treatment by those in charge of her medical care, we would like to go ahead and give her suggestions that would benefit her immediately.

The patient was counseled extensively at the end of the final testing session, which was attended by her friend. This friend, also a nun in charge of the patient's religious duties, was very helpful in coming up with solutions. As with many patients, with the help of her friend, she was able to arrive at many of the solutions to her dangerous activities herself.

We made an informal sketch of her apartment and found several problem areas, including a side door to the outside with steps without a railing through which she frequently brings groceries and other items. She told us that the apartment manager would not make any changes to her apartment, but that many safety items such as grab bars in the bathroom were already installed. Unfortunately, there were several areas in the apartment where the level changed with a single step between rooms. The friend assured us that other safety features would be installed such as rails at key locations in the apartment where the level changed. The dangerous side door without the rail remained a problem because it seemed no rail would be possible and it was the closest to the car to bring groceries through. After discussing this problem, the patient finally decided that a solution would be to use the back door for bringing items in. A basket with wheels would be used to transport the items the greater distance to the back door. This cart would also help to stabilize the patient while walking, whereas carrying the groceries as previously without support only added to the danger.

One by one, the patient and her friend worked out a solution to each problem situation. By discussing in detail each area of the patient's living quarters and each daily habit, workable solutions were arrived at. Perhaps the most interesting problem to be worked out involved the religious ritual that required the patient to carry the heavy prayer book up to the front of the chapel during worship services. This was a sensitive subject for the patient because it had been her tradition to be honored to perform this duty for several years. Tears came to her eyes at the prospect of not being able to perform this religious task any longer. That is when the friend came to the rescue. Being the religious superior to the patient, the friend suggested that perhaps someone could accompany her in carrying the book up to the front of the chapel and that this would be acceptable modification to the religious ritual. This successfully solved the patient's dilemma to her satisfaction. Without the accompanying friend, an entirely different outcome might have resulted. It was difficult for the patient to agree to any life-changing modifications but when she was helped to see that these changes would not affect her lifestyle significantly, she gladly accepted them.

What We Learned

Although the standard recommendation for this patient would have been to use a walker, it was apparent that the patient was unwilling to accept this. Instead, modifications to the apartment were recommended that included more furniture, rails, and other accommodations that would result in a living space that would not have any open areas without something to hold onto. Her religious duties were modified just enough to make them safe but without changing their basic manner or significance.

Case 6

Principle Demonstrated in This Case

For some older individuals, not much can be done to prevent further falls but some measures can be taken to prevent injury once falls occur. These situations stem from the unfortunate combination of factors of there not being a medical "cure" for the problem as well as the patient's unwillingness to use assistive walking devices or comply with other recommendations to prevent falls.

This situation may also be true of frail older individuals who have nothing particularly "wrong" with their balance systems as far as testing goes, but do have the changes associated with normal aging such as lowered sensitivity in the sensory and motor balance systems, weakened muscle strength, slower reaction speeds, and mildly slowed cognitive function. In such cases, the emphasis may need to shift toward injury prevention because the measures suggested to simply prevent injuries may be more acceptable to the patient.

The Problem

Mr. K., a healthy looking 88-year-old who lives with his healthy 80-year-old wife, has few medical problems other than osteoporosis and controlled anemia, but experiences falls about every other month. He broke his left hip 2 years ago in a fall in which he was coming out of a bathroom stall and fell backward. Falls occur without feelings of dizziness, imbalance, or weakness and occur while walking with no identifiable pattern respecting falls circumstances. He does not tend to fall when first standing up. Many recent falls that he describes occur when he is going up or down a single step such as a curb or going down the single step leading from his back walk to his driveway. He has also recently fallen when after standing, he began to walk again while turning to the right. He may also fall after bending over, while carrying things, or at other random times.

Results of Testing

Abnormal Results

The only abnormal result of the falls screening evaluation was a mildly unsteady gait attributed to a slight weakness in the left hip area, the previously broken hip. Although he easily passes the strength screenings for ankles, knees, and hips, he describes "heaviness in both legs for the past several years," and says that his left leg is somewhat less responsive or weak, which he feels stems from his previous broken hip. On the strength screening, there is only a slight left hip weakness in the abductor and adductor muscles compared to the right. He exercises regularly using weights and is noticeably stronger than average in the lower extremities for his age.

He can stand on foam for a few seconds with eyes closed then falls backward consistently. This is probably within normal limits for his age and represents only a mild vestibular decrement in sensory function.

He performs normally on the Romberg, tandem Romberg, and Tinetti test of informal balance function. His contrast vision, cognition, and mood are normal. He is not orthostatic. He complains of no numbness of the lower extremities.

Evaluation of his living surroundings was made by sketching the floor plan and discussing his daily and weekly habits in relation to his surroundings. It was discovered that the patient has adequate furniture to hold onto for making trips to the bathroom at night (once per night) but that there is a lack of rails on the front and back steps outside the home. The patient also has no portable or cell phone, although he makes frequent trips outside the home alone.

Results Summary

The patient has mild decrement in sensory and/or motor balance due to normal aging processes. This is termed "presbystasis." Due to the past falls, the patient is at high risk for future falls, which are expected to occur at about the same frequency. There is high risk of further injury if no intervention is made. There is a particular risk of the patient falling in the backward direction, although falls also occur in any direction.

Solutions

The results just noted in the Results Summary were explained to the patient, with the admonition that, although the patient is in excellent health and physical condition, there is high likelihood of continued falls and probable injury if changes are not made.

The following recommendations were made:

1. Install handrails on the stairs.
2. Obtain a cell phone or alerting device.

What We Learned

Some people's falls are likely to continue due to medical problems that cannot be solved, behavioral issues, or a combination of the two. Sometimes the only thing to do is work on making the surroundings safer so that, when falls do occur, there will be less chance of injury. There should also be some type of alerting device or someone should check on the person regularly.

Conclusion

No two falls cases are the same. It is beneficial to try to arrive at the most important falls cause in each individual, remembering that sometimes this will be a behavioral issue. Finding the right solution will also be an individual matter that requires an interview with the patient regarding the environmental factors involved.

Suggested Additional Readings on Gait

Craik, R. (1995). *Gait analysis: Theory and application*. St. Louis, MO: Mosby.

DeLisa, J. A. (1998). *Gait analysis in the science of rehabilitation*. Washington, DC: Department of Veterans Affairs, Veterans Health Administration.

Inman, V. T., Ralston, H. J., & Todd, F. (1981). *Human walking*. Baltimore: Williams & Wilkins.

Perry, J. (1992). *Gait analysis: Normal and pathological function*. Thorofare, NJ: SLACK.

Rose J., & Gamble J. G. (1994). *Human walking* (2nd ed.). Baltimore: Williams & Wilkins.

Sutherland, D. H. (1989). *The development of mature walking*. Oxford, UK: Blackwell.

Vaughan, C. L., Davis, B. L., & O'Connor, J. (1992). *Dynamics of human gait*. Champaign, IL: Human Kinetics.

Vaughan, C. L., Davis, B. L., & O'Connor, J. (1999). *Dynamics of human gait* (2nd ed.). Cape Town, South Africa: Kiboho.

Whittle, M. (1991). *Gait analysis: An introduction*. Boston: Butterworth-Heinemann.

Winter, D. A. (1990). *Biomechanics and motor control of human movement* (2nd ed.). New York: Wiley.

Winter, D. A. (1991). *The biomechanics and motor control of human gait: Normal, elderly and pathological* (2nd ed.). Waterloo, Ontario: University of Waterloo Press.

Winter, D. A. (1995). *A.B.C. (anatomy, biomechanics and control) of balance during standing and walking*. Waterloo, Ontario: Waterloo Biomechanics.

APPENDIX B

Example Falls Clinic Reports and Sample Blank Forms

Example 1: Falls Prevention Clinic Report

Patient: Example patient
Date:

History

For the past 5 years, the patient complains of pressure in the head with dizziness when rising or moving his head quickly side to side. He is not vertiginous and feels no dizziness when sitting or lying. He also complains of becoming tired easily. Symptoms become better in the afternoon or evening. He had a mastoidectomy on the right many years ago. He has high frequency hearing loss L>R for many years which is stable. The ENT is currently reviewing the recent MRI with the otologist, which is pending.

Medical conditions pertinent to falls

CVA in 1975, essential tremors since 7 to 8 years which are stable, coronary artery disease with past bypass grafting, vasovagal sensitivity.

Medications possibly contributing to falls include:

Florinef, Zoloft, Namenda, ReQuip, Sanctura, Avandia, Zelnorm, Pravachol, Lyrica, Lunestra, Nexium.

Examination:

Vestibular and balance testing:

Overall results are consistent with two abnormal conditions, namely,

1. Uncompensated vestibulopathy, nonlocalizing as shown by a transient nystagmus produced on lateral head shaking for 30 seconds (right beating, 5 deg/sec decreasing to zero in 10 seconds). For this, the patient had been given self-directed vesitbular rehabilitation exercises at the previous visit, which he reports he is performing.

2. The second abnormal condition is **abnormal postural responses** possibly representing a movement disorder rather than a sensory balance system disorder. This is demonstrated by abnormal scores on the Motor Control Test portion of the posturography examination, in which he exhibited slow reactions to sudden platform perturbations. Consistent with this finding were the informal balance tests. He could barely stand on thick foam with his eyes open without falling. This is a central nervous system sign as opposed to a vestibular sign, as he was no worse with eyes closed.

3. Other informal balance tests were consistent with a general unsteadiness when walking especially when turning and more consistent with a movement related disorder than a sensory balance system disorder. He nearly fell when turning quickly during the Up and Go test although his time was normal (10 seconds). He was also very unsteady when turning a small circle in place with eyes open. On the marching Fukuda test, he did not deviate to either side, but it was difficult for him to perform the marching movement at all with eyes closed.

The rest of the formal balance function testing was normal. VNG, and Rotational Chair testing showed robust symmetrical vestibular responses to caloric and rotational chair testing respectively. Posturography today was normal for vestibular, somatosensory, and visual static standing balance, although automatic postural responses were abnormal.

Orthostatic blood pressure:

Lying 5 min: 123/78 P-73, Standing: 111/76 P-83 Normal

Vision:

Normal acuity and contrast vision (acuity binocular best corrected – 20/30, Melborn Edges test (contrast vision) <19 Normal)

Lower extremities strength and feeling:

Normal strength (5/5) for ankles, knees, and hips bilaterally, but abnormal feeling as previously diagnosed in feet and lower legs bilaterally.

Reaction times:

Normal for hand (277 msec ave) and foot (210 msec)

Summary/Recommendations

On the positive side, the patient has quite normal scores for orthostatics, strength in the lower extremities, vision, and reaction times.

Things to check into:

1. Two distinct types of balance abnormalities were suggested by test results. Primarily, several test results were consistent with a **movement-related balance** deficit (see above). This is manifested in a practical sense by instability and near falls whenever he is walking or turning quickly. In addition, there is evidence of an **uncompensated vestibulopathy** (see above), which is probably of less importance. Self-directed vestibular rehabilitation exercises were given to the patient for this latter deficit.
2. Previously diagnosed peripheral neuropathy causing some difficulty sensing the ground with his feet.

Physical therapy is not recommended; rather, the patient was instructed to follow up with his primary physician as some of the medications he is on have the capability of producing dizziness and/or imbalance.

If you have any questions, please feel free to contact me,

Sincerely,

Lynn S. Alvord
Falls Clinic Director
(phone number)

Example 2: Falls Clinic Report

Patient:

History

After walking, her right leg feels weak. She occasionally falls and stumbles. She feels no dizziness except when get up fast.

Medical problems pertinent to falls include:

>   **Vestibular (Overall results):** Abnormal left peripheral vestibular disorder (see recent Balance Function Test report)

>   **Orthostatic hypotension:** Abnormal (BP 140/80 lying; 115/75 standing)

>   **Peripheral neuropathy:** Abnormal to light touch, pin prick, and tuning fork bilaterally

>   **Vision:** Normal visual acuity, binocular corrected 20/20. Normal contrast vision

>   **Lower extremity strength:** Low strength bilaterally for ankles, knee and hips (4/5)

Results/Recommendations

On the positive side:

You have excellent vision, including vision for contrast. You have no complaints or signs of abnormal cognition or mood.

Things to check into:

From recent tests, your falling is likely due to a combination of the following:

>   a. Drop in blood pressure when first standing
>   b. Inner ear "dizziness"

c. Weakness in the legs

d. Reduced feeling in the legs and feet

Follow up with your primary doctor and Ear, Nose, and Throat doctor for these problems

Particular risky situations for you include:

When reaching up, when getting back up such as after picking something up, turning while walking, walking when outside the house, in the dark or on soft surfaces. Don't walk outside alone.

Below is a list of suggestions specifically for you to help prevent further falls:

1. Go to your ENT physician concerning the inner ear problem that causes you to be dizzy
2. Get a "grabber" for picking up things off the floor and from upper shelves
3. Consider changing bedroom locations to the main floor
4. Hold on when first standing (say a poem)
5. Install handrail for front porch steps
6. Grab bars for the bathroom
7. More furniture to hold onto
8. Get rid of throw rug in bedroom
9. Carry portable phone at all times
10. Use steps one at a time. Go up with the strong leg first (left) and down with the weak leg first (right)
11. Use a cane or walker as recommended by a physical therapist
12. Don't use a new kind of shoes you are not used to
13. Review the items on the checklist handout provided
14. Bifocals or reading glasses cause significant problems with persons having a tendency to fall because looking toward the floor through the lower portion of the bifocals or reading glasses causes distortion of the ground which often causes falls. Inability to see the ground or the feet properly is a common factor leading to falls.
15. There is need for nightlights because you perform much worse in the dark and on soft surfaces, as is the case on carpet at night traveling to the bathroom. A bedside commode could also be considered.

16. You were counseled regarding the risk of rushing to the phone or door.
17. Your living environment should also be checked for safety features to prevent falls. I spoke to you about these issues and gave you a brochure of home safety features. Please review these.
18. You are expected to be at most risk in darkened environments and on soft surfaces.

If there are any further questions, please feel free to contact me.

Sincerely,

Lynn S. Alvord
Falls Clinic Director
(phone number)

Example 3: Falls Clinic Report

Patient:

History

The patient feels off-balance after walking awhile.

Medical problems previously diagnosed include:

Two heart attacks in recent years, anemia, arrhythmia, and hypertension.

Examination

Vestibular tests:

Bilateral vestibular weakness by formal testing (see report of 9/1/2006). Informal balance testing shows that the patient is off-balance nearly falling when turning a small circle in place. He cannot march with eyes closed.

Lower extremity strength:

Normal 4/5 or 5/5 for ankles, hips, knees bilaterally

Lower extremity sensation:

Normal to pin-prick, and tuning fork to big toe bilaterally. Proprioception is normal for big toe up or down.

Vision:

20/70 ABNORMAL

Orthostatics:

Abnormal. The patient is hypotensive, BP lying = 156/77, P-74 BP standing = 135/71, P-81

Environment and Habits:

Patient lives alone next door to his granddaughter.

Results/Recommendations

On the positive side:

1. You are very strong and coordinated
2. You are mentally sharp
3. You will be improving your hearing on Friday by the use of your new hearing aids
4. You have good feeling in your feet and legs

Things to check into for improvement:

1. Vision (20/70 and abnormal contrast vision)
2. Blood pressure drops when standing (hold on for 1 minute before walking, poem)
3. Getting used to your new hearing aid that you will be issued on Friday will be a positive step to your socialization. In order to help in your adjustment, try the following with the help of a family member: Go to the store once per week, a friend or relative's once per week, church or social gathering once per week

Other things to consider:

1. There is need for night lights because you will have much worse balance in the dark or on soft surfaces, as is the case on carpet at night traveling to the bathroom. A bedside commode could also be considered.
2. There is risk of falling when rushing to the phone or door.
3. Your living environment should also be checked for safety features to prevent falls. I spoke to you regarding these safety issues and gave you a brochure of home safety features. Please review these.

If there are any further questions, please feel free to contact me.

Sincerely,

Lynn S. Alvord
Falls Clinic Director
(phone number)

Falls Clinic Results of Individual Tests (data sheet)

This form is used only to collect test data during the Falls Clinic visits. The Final Report template is shown following this template

Patient name: **Date of Test:**

Referred by: **Referral date:**

History (Pertinent Past/Current Medical History, Falls History):

How many falls have you had in the past 6 months? _____
past 1 month? _____

What were the circumstances of those falls?

Environmental factors:

Medications affecting balance/vertigo/dizziness:

   Past ototoxic medications:

Balance function tests (formal):

   Overall Results:

Results of individual tests:

   VNG: **Rotational Chair:**   **Hallpike:**

   Posturography: Informal Balance Evaluation:

                       Romberg:

                       Tandem Romberg:

                       Fukuda:

Tinneti:

Gait:

Up and Go test:

Cognitive function/Mood:

Orthostatic BP: **Lying 5 min:**   **Standing:**

Peripheral neuropathy screen:

Vision:

Lower muscle strength:

  Knee flexion/extension:

  Ankle flexion/extension:

  Hip flexion/extension:

Physical Therapy Evaluation Results:

Summary/Recommendations:

History for Vestibular (Balance Function) Testing

Name:

Date:

MRN:

1. Describe your dizziness, balance disorder, or lightheaded complaint:

2. When did you first notice the symptoms? _____ Had they happened before that (for example, years ago?) _____

3. Are your symptoms truly episodic, that is, are you always a little bit dizzy (lightheaded, etc.) or are there days at a time that you are completely free of these symptoms?

4. What would your problem most accurately be called (circle only one):
   a. Lightheadedness   b. Spinning   c. Off-balance

5. Is there anything that causes your symptoms to occur or make them worse? (referring to your feeling of either "off balance", dizziness or lightheadedness)

6. Do you recall the first time you felt the symptoms?

7. Did the symptoms come on suddenly or gradually?

8. Was the first episode the worst?

9. If the first was not the worst, were the first couple of episodes the worst ones?

10. Are these symptoms getting worse, getting gradually better or about the same as they were in the beginning?

11. Are your symptoms either made to occur or made worse by (circle all that apply):
    a. Moving quickly? (which direction?)
    b. Moving your head side to side
    c. Looking up
    d. Coming up after bending over
    e. While bending over
    f. Lying down
    g. Getting up from lying down
    h. Rolling over in bed (which direction?)
    i. In the dark
    j. When you cough or sneeze
    k. When you lift or bear down such as going to the bathroom
    l. When you sing, yell, or speak loudly
    m. When you hear loud sounds
    n. Exercise
    o. Walking a long way
    p. First getting up from sitting
    q. Other (list anything you do that makes your symptoms worse)

12. Referring to the question above, circle three or four of the worst ones (the ones which make your dizziness the worst).

13. Is there a time of day that you have more of your symptoms?

14. Do you ever have your symptoms when: (circle those that apply)
    a. Standing without walking
    b. sitting
    c. lying down
    d. standing when walking

15. Do you get any *other symptoms* along with your dizziness (at about the same time)? (circle those that apply)
    a. headache
    b. flashes of light in your vision
    c. sensitivity to sounds
    d. weakness
    e. numbness
    f. confusion
    g. faint feeling
    h. difficulty speaking
    i. accidental urination or defecation
    j. falls
    k. heart palpitations or racing pulse
    l. loss of consciousness

16. Any medications that may affect the test (pain pills, "dizzy pills," tranquilizers, sleeping pills)?

Falls Clinic Report

[name of clinic]

[address of clinic]

(This report is a summary of **<u>abnormal</u>** test results from the Falls Clinic visit. For more detailed results of individual tests including all normal results, see "Falls Clinic Results of Individual Tests," See also results of Balance Function Testing which includes detailed results of VNG, Rotational Chair-which are scanned into the medical record)

Patient:

Date:

Balance and Falls Complaints:

Number of falls in the past 6 months:

Number of falls in the past month:

Injuries with falls:

Circumstances of falls:

Past pertinent medical history:

Medications possibly causing falls:

Results

Vestibular:

Posturography results:

Sensory organization test:

    Composite Score:

        Abnormal Patterns:

        Somatosensory: YES/NO

        Visual: YES/NO

        Vestibular: YES/NO

Motor control test:

Adaptation test:

VNG/ENG Results (summary):

Rotational Chair Results:

VEMPS Results:

Summary Vestibular Results:

Orthostatic/cardiogenic (known/suspected at this visit):

Medical/metabolic disorder (known/suspected at this visit):

Neurological disorder (known/suspected at this visit):

Medications review (possibly affecting balance):

Lower extremity weakness/neuropathy (known/suspected at this visit):

Visual (known/suspected at this visit):

Cognition/mood:

Environmental/ lifestyle risk factors:

Other abnormal risk factors thought to be less contributory to the

patient's falls/balance problem:

Informal (bedside) tests for gait, balance, and falls risk

Summary/Recommendations:

On the positive side:

1. List strengths of the patient for preventing falls (good strength in the lower extremities, etc.)
2. and so forth.

Items for follow-up:

1. List items to be followed up on to prevent falls (test abnormalities, recommendations for physical therapy, behavior modifications, rearranging items in the home, etc.
2. Consult with your primary doctor regarding medications that may be affecting your blood pressure.
3. and so forth.

In summary, the patient is considered at (medium or high) risk for falling. Consider fall-proofing the home by removing loose rugs, installing grab bars, installing carpeting on floor where there is none to cushion falls, as well as implementing the other suggestions in the handout. The results were discussed with the patient including home safety issues.

APPENDIX C

Safety Checklist

(large letters for easy reading by aging patients)

Safety Checklist for
Avoiding Falls in Your Home

Stairways

Install handrails at all stairways
  Do the handrails support a person's weight?

Keep floors and steps clear of clutter

Throw away "throw rugs"

Use colored tape at the top and bottom of stairs
  to identify the first and last step

Good lighting at all locations in the house,
  especially for use at night

Bathroom

Install grab bars near bathtub, shower, and toilet

Keep soap in the soap holder

Place nonslip rubber mats in the bathtub and
  shower.

Nonskid rug outside the bathtub to dry feet

Elevated toilet seats or handles

Bedside commode

Family Room, Bedroom, and Kitchen

Wipe up spills

Use floor wax that is slip-resistant.

Wait for floors to dry after cleaning

Avoid cords, oxygen tubing, and other hazards in pathways.

Place commonly used items in easy to reach

Do not use stepladders or stools to stand on (use a long-handled "reacher" or rearrange objects to lower shelves

Avoid chairs having wheels

Chairs should have arm rests for easy exiting

When rising, stand slowly if dizziness occurs, and regain balance before walking.

Use automatic on/off night-lights to light pathways

Always keep a charged flashlight and telephone in your bedrooms for emergencies

Carry a portable phone or safety alert

APPENDIX D

Alvord Falls Screening Test

Patient name:
Dob:
Date:

		Yes	No
History:	Previous falls? (2 or more in one year, or 1 if injury)	☐	☐
	Medications that are affecting patient's performance? (subjective rating by examiner)	☐	☐
	Room spins?	☐	☐
	Knees give out causing falls?	☐	☐
Vestibular:	Nearly falls when walking while turning head?	☐	☐
	Falls soon when standing on thick foam, with eyes open or closed?	☐	☐
	Abnormal Dix-Hallpike test?	☐	☐
Lower extremities:	Reduced strength or feeling	☐	☐
	Significant pain or weakness when walking?	☐	☐
Psych/Behavioral:	Dementia?	☐	☐
	Depression?	☐	☐
	Risky habits (rushing, carrying on stairs, etc.)?	☐	☐
Cardiovascular:	Orthostatic hypotension?	☐	☐
	Irregular pulse or palpitations or other heart disease that cause symptoms?	☐	☐
Neurologic:	Stroke, Parkinson's or other neurologic disorder that affects movements?	☐	☐
Informal balance:	"Up and Go test" abnormal (nearly falls or >20 seconds)	☐	☐
	Unsteady gait?	☐	☐

		Yes	No
	Tinetti abnormal—unsteady when turns in circle in place, when nudged, turning in place, reaching high, picking up, using stairs?	☐	☐
	Functional reach—falls reaching less than 12 inches?	☐	☐
Vision:	Vision corrected is 20/50 or worse binocular	☐	☐
Other:	Other obvious risk factor?		

Pass/Fail:

Comments:

INDEX